Study Guide for the
Core Curriculum for Oncology Nursing

EDITED BY

CLAUDETTE G. VARRICCHIO, DSN, RN, OCN, FAAN

Associate Professor
Niehoff School of Nursing
Loyola University, Chicago
Chicago, Illinois

PATRICIA F. JASSAK, MS, RN, CS, OCN

Oncology Clinical Nurse Specialist
Foster G. McGaw Hospital
Loyola University Medical Center
Maywood, Illinois
Clinical Assistant Professor
Niehoff School of Nursing
Loyola University, Chicago
Chicago, Illinois

W.B. SAUNDERS COMPANY

Harcourt Brace Jovanovich, Inc.

Philadelphia • London • Toronto • Montreal • Sydney • Tokyo

W.B. SAUNDERS COMPANY
Harcourt Brace Jovanovich, Inc.

The Curtis Center
Independence Square West
Philadelphia, Pennsylvania 19106

Editor: Thomas Eoyang

STUDY GUIDE FOR THE CORE CURRICULUM
FOR ONCOLOGY NURSING

ISBN   0–7216–3487–7

Printed in Mexico

Last digit is the print number: 9   8   7   6   5   4   3   2

Contributors

KAREN L. FITZ ADELMAN, RN, BS, OCN

M. D. Anderson Cancer Center
University of Texas
Houston, Texas
Genitourinary

ANNE E. BELCHER, PhD, RN

University of Maryland School of Nursing
Baltimore, Maryland
*Informed Consent, Legislation and Ethics; and Cancer
Through the Life Span*

CATHERINE M. BENDER, RN, MN

University of Pittsburgh
Pittsburgh, Pennsylvania
Chemotherapy

JANICE BESCHORNER, RN, MS, OCN

University of Chicago Hospitals
Chicago, Illinois
Biological Response Modifiers

KAREN SMITH BLESCH, RN, MS

Central Dupage Hospital
Winfield, Illinois
Cancer Epidemiology

JENNIFER DUNN BUCHOLTZ, RN, MS

University of Delaware
Department of Advanced Nursing Science
The Johns Hopkins University School of Nursing
Baltimore, Maryland
Radiation

JANE C. CLARK, MN, RN, OCN

Emory University Hospital
Atlanta, Georgia
*Nursing Management of Responses to the Cancer
Experience*

KATHY COYLE, RN, BSN

Bone Marrow Transplant Unit
Shands Hospital
University of Florida
Gainesville, Florida
Bone Marrow Transplantation

MARY CUNNINGHAM, RN, MS

University of Texas School of Nursing
Department of Neuro-oncology
M. D. Anderson Cancer Center
Houston, Texas
*Standards of Practice and Education; and
Professional Issues*

LEONITA H. CUTRIGHT, RN, MSN

Memorial Hospital
Chattanooga, Tennessee
Head and Neck

MARILYN DAVIS, RN, MS

Medical and Scientific Affairs Department
Schering-Plough Corporation
Kenilworth, New Jersey
*Cancer Prevention and Detection; and
Biological Response Modifiers*

EILEEN McQUAID DVORAK, PhD, RN

Niehoff School of Nursing
Loyola University, Chicago
Chicago, Illinois
Overview of Testing

NINA M. ENTREKIN, RN, MN, OCN

Breast Cancer Task Force
American Cancer Society Florida Division, Inc.
H. Lee Moffitt Cancer Center
Tampa, Florida
Breast

LYNN ERDMAN, RN, MN, OCN

Presbyterian Hospital
Charlotte, North Carolina
Supportive Therapies and Procedures

MARIE FLANNERY, RN, MS

University of Rochester Cancer Center and School of
Nursing
Rochester, New York
Reproductive

MARILYN FRANK-STROMBORG, RN, EdD,
FAAN

Northern Illinois University
De Kalb, Illinois
Cancer Prevention and Detection; and Cancer Epidemiology

CATHY L. GRACE-LOUTHEN, RN, MSN, OCN

Humana Hospital–Michael Reese
Chicago, Illinois
Surgery

JAMES P. HALLORAN, MSN, RN, OCN, ANP

Association of Nurses in AIDS Care
University of Texas School of Public Health
HIV Infection and AIDS

JANE C. HUNTER, RN, MN, OCN

Presbyterian Hospital Cancer Center
Charlotte, North Carolina
Oncologic Emergencies

LINDA LEAH HUNTER, MS, RN, OCN, ET

Formerly of H. Lee Moffitt Cancer Center
Tampa, Florida
Professional Issues

JUDITH L. JOHNSON, RN, PhD

University of Minnesota School of Nursing
North Memorial Medical Center
Minneapolis, Minnesota
Standards of Practice and Education

MARY B. JOHNSON, RN, PhD, OCN

St. Olaf College
Minnesota Intercollegiate Nursing Consortium
Abbott Northwestern Hospital
Minneapolis, Minnesota
Standards of Practice and Education

NANCY E. KANE, RN, MS, OCN

Catholic Medical Center
Manchester, New Hampshire
Unproven Methods

TONI KLATT-ELLIS, RN, MN

University of South Bend
Memorial Hospital
South Bend, Indiana
Informed Consent, Legislation and Ethics

MARILYN A. KLINE, RN, BSN, OCN

Tucson, Arizona
Oncologic Emergencies

TRACY KRESEK, BSN, RN

Memorial Sloan-Kettering Cancer Center
New York, New York
Sarcoma

LOIS J. LOESCHER, MS, RN

University of Arizona Cancer Center
Tucson, Arizona
Survivorship

ALICE J. LONGMAN, EdD, RN, FAAN

University of Arizona
College of Nursing
Tucson, Arizona
Skin

CATHY MAZZONE, RN, MS, OCN

University of Maryland School of Nursing
University of Maryland Cancer Center
Hematologic and Lymphatic Systems

ROSE F. McGEE, PhD, RN

Nell Hodgson Woodruff School of Nursing
Emory University
Atlanta, Georgia
*Nursing Management of Responses to the Cancer
Experience*

DEBORAH STEPHENS MILLS, RN, MN, OCN

Holston Valley Hospital and Medical Center
Christine LaGuardia Phillips Cancer Center
Kingsport, Tennessee
Care Settings

BETTY M. OWENS, BA, BSN, MS

University of Colorado
Health Sciences Center
Division of Neurosurgery
Denver, Colorado
Neurologic

LISA POTANOVICH, RN, BSN

Memorial Sloan-Kettering Cancer Center
New York, New York
Lung

FREDRICA A. PRESTON, RN, MA

Formerly of Hospital of the University of Pennsylvania
Philadelphia, Pennsylvania
*Nursing Management of Responses to the Cancer
Experience*

MARCIA E. ROSTAD, RN, MS, NS, OCN

College of Nursing
University of Arizona
University Medical Center
Tucson, Arizona
Supportive Therapies and Procedures

ROBERTA ANNE STROHL, RN, MN

University of Maryland at Baltimore
Baltimore, Maryland
Gastro-intestinal

THOMAS J. SZOPA, MS, RN, OCN, CETN

University of New Hampshire
Durham, New Hampshire
Elliot Hospital
Manchester, New Hampshire
Surgery

LINDA TENENBAUM, RN, MSN, OCN

Department of Nursing
Broward Community College
Fort Lauderdale, Florida
Chemotherapy

LESLIE B. TYSON, BSN

Memorial Sloan-Kettering Cancer Center
New York, New York
Supportive Therapies and Procedures; and Lung

DEBORAH L. VOLKER, RN, MA, OCN

M. D. Anderson Cancer Center
University of Texas
Houston, Texas
*Standards of Practice and Education; Pathophysiology of
Cancer: General Concepts; and The Process of
Carcinogenesis*

Reviewers

TERRY CHAMORRO, RN, MN, CS, OCN

Cedars-Sinai Medical Center
Los Angeles, California

APRIL J. DUMOND, RN, MSN, OCN

Arkansas Cancer Research Center
Little Rock, Arkansas

JOY L. FINCANNON, MS, RN, OCN, CS

The Johns Hopkins Oncology Center
Baltimore, Maryland

CATHY GRACE-LOUTHEN, RN, BSN, OCN

Humana Hospital–Michael Reese
Chicago, Illinois

RYAN R. IWAMOTO, RN, MN, CS

Virginia Mason Clinic
Seattle, Washington

M. TISH KNOBF, RN, MSN, FAAN

Yale University School of Nursing
New Haven, Connecticut

PATRICIA E. LAWLER, RN, MS

Lutheran General Hospital
Park Ridge, Illinois

MARY BETH RILEY, RN, MSN, OCN

Arkansas Cancer Research Center
Little Rock, Arkansas

CHRISTINE L. QUIRCH, RN, BSN, OCN

Loyola University Medical Center
Maywood, Illinois

JOANN F. PETTY, RN, MSN, OCN,

Loyola University Medical Center
Maywood, Illinois

NANCY L. PORTER, MS, RN, OCN

Loyola University Medical Center
Maywood, Illinois

JOANNE REIFSNYDER, RN, MSN, OCN

Thomas Jefferson University
Philadelphia, Pennsylvania

ELLEN ROTH, RN, MSN

Northwestern Memorial Hospital
Chicago, Illinois

ELIZABETH J. SANTAS, RN, BSN, OCN

Loyola University Chicago
Chicago, Illinois

SANDRA LEE SCHAFER, RN, MN, OCN

Shadyside Hospital
Pittsburgh, Pennsylvania

Preface

The *Study Guide for the Core Curriculum for Oncology Nursing*, a companion to the *Core Curriculum for Oncology Nursing*, is a resource for nurses who want to review a basic level of oncology nursing knowledge and for those who want to assess their knowledge in this area. This book may also serve as a reference source of information on oncology nursing topics. Educators may find it useful as a bank of test questions to guide the development of course related materials.

This book is based on, and intended to be a companion volume to, the *Core Curriculum for Oncology Nursing*, 2nd edition. Many of the questions, rationales and references were prepared by the authors of the corresponding section of the *Core Curriculum*. All of the questions and rationales were reviewed by oncology nurses, often OCNs, for clinical relevance, accuracy, consistency with current practice, and clarity. The items were also reviewed for technical test item construction by Eileen McQuaid Dvorak, an expert in test item writing, and former Executive Director, National Council of State Boards of Nursing.

The book is divided into chapters whose content parallels the *Core Curriculum*. Each chapter has multiple choice questions. The correct answer and a rationale for the answer are provided. The *Core Curriculum for Oncology Nursing*, 2nd edition, is the primary source for the text. A list of additional references is given at the end of each chapter for the material covered in that section.

The number of questions on each topic was derived from the percent of questions for that content area established by the Oncology Nursing Certification Corporation in the "Blueprint for the Oncology Nursing Certification Exam" provided to applicants for the certification exam. The subjects covered in both this study guide and in the *Core Curriculum* go beyond those known to be included in the certification exam.

The *Study Guide for the Core Curriculum for Oncology Nursing* has many potential uses. It is one of many ways to meet the challenges presented by the professional practice of oncology nursing.

CLAUDETTE G. VARRICCHIO
PATRICIA F. JASSAK

Acknowledgments

The editors wish to acknowledge the Oncology Nursing Society and the Education Committee for their support in the initiation and development of this project. Special thanks are extended to item writer colleagues who spent many hours diligently preparing test questions. We also thank the item reviewers who critiqued the questions. We wish to especially acknowledge Arlene Knop for her superb secretarial and organizational assistance in the preparation of the manuscript in its final form.

Contents

12
Characteristics of Major Cancers

1
Overview of Testing

Eileen McQuaid Dvorak

Preparation for the Test

Testing is a method used to evaluate a person's knowledge, skill, and/or ability in a specific area. The purpose of the evaluation may be for self-information, for recognition by peers or others, or for entrance to a specific profession or occupation. Certification testing is used to recognize a person's special knowledge of a particular field or segment thereof.

Many varieties of tests exist. These can be multiple-choice, essay, completion, simulation, or performance. Most commonly, for testing large numbers of people, a multiple-choice question format is used. Use of this format expedites the processing of results and, more importantly, permits testing a broader range of a person's abilities. Knowing the type of questions or format of a particular test will help you prepare a strategy to ease the stress inherent in taking any test. In this book the format used is multiple-choice.

There is also a variety of forms of administration of tests; paper-and-pencil, computerized, oral, laboratory, or clinical demonstration are common. Currently the most common form is paper-and-pencil testing. Knowing the format of administration also helps you to prepare a test-taking strategy. As an example, if you take certain computerized examinations, you may not return to a question previously skipped. In certain patient simulation formats, selection of one answer necessitates following specific directions to other tracks of questioning. In a paper-and-pencil test, unlike a computerized one, you can return to questions skipped. One should attempt to answer all questions as directed regardless of format.

Review

One of the first steps in preparing for a test is to obtain the content outline of the examination from the certifying organization. This "blueprint" is a primary source of information for the examination. The outline also gives the priority of each section by identifying the weight or percentage of questions for each specific part of the examination. Knowing the general content and priority established will help guide your review of content by correlating the examination emphasis with your confidence in your knowledge of that section.

Once the content and priority of the sections are known, you can schedule review time and find source material. If bibliographies are provided by the sponsoring body, use the references suggested. These are probably the ones provided by the experts who wrote the test questions or who decided on the content outline.

As mentioned before, review the content outline and focus your preparation on those areas where you feel less confident. Many certification examinations test one's ability to apply knowledge. In your review, test yourself concerning facts or principles and how you apply these in your practice.

How you review the test material depends on your personal style or preference. Some people prefer to work alone and pace their review according to their needs. Other persons prefer to work in a group and learn from the process of questioning one another and conferring with others about areas where questions exist. Still others prefer a combination of individual and group review. No one way is best. If you do plan to work with a group, either totally or sometimes, make certain all

1

members agree in advance on the content to be covered at each session and the time of the meetings. Verifying the group's agenda and expectations in advance will offset future conflicts if some members later think their individual needs are not being met in the group sessions.

Another important part of review is to try test questions in advance. The questions in this book are similar in design and overall content to those used in certification examinations. Try them to help determine areas where you need more concentrated review. After reviewing the questions, check the content areas and consider the knowledge being tested; this will give you direction for your continued review. Another outcome of trying the test questions in this book is that you will learn to pace yourself. The first time you take the questions, time yourself. More on pacing the test is contained in the next section.

The amount of time needed to prepare for the examination is another individual matter. Only you can determine how much content you need to review or how secure you feel about your knowledge in each area. People involved in test development recommend that you not study immediately before an examination, because you will be under the stress that comes from knowing that your knowledge, skill, and ability are going to be evaluated. Studying the night before an exam increases that stress. Try to find some diversion. Consider exercising—exercise does relieve anxiety. Try some means of exercising the evening or morning before an exam to help "burn off" the excess adrenalin.

Writing the Test

One of the most important points to remember in taking any test is to read the directions. It sounds simplistic to say it, but many astute, knowledgeable practitioners score poorly on examinations because they do not read the instructions. If you do not understand a direction, contact someone from the certifying organization and ask for an explanation. This is not a reading comprehension test. You have a right to understand fully what direction is being given, so do not hesitate to ask for assistance in this regard.

Once you have started taking the test, pace yourself. Generally, in multiple-choice questions, the writers have estimated that it will take one minute per question. Some obviously take less time; some may take more. But, one minute per question is the average. If you do not know the answer to a question after carefully reading it, go on to the next one and make a note to return to that number. I have found that you can categorize these "unknowns" into those questions about which you have some idea of the content and those in which the content is totally unknown to you. Put the questions into these two categories to save time when you return to respond to them. Reconsider first those which you had an idea about the content, and then spend your final testing time on those totally unknown to you.

It is important not to make these lists on the test answer sheet; use your test booklet. Do not mark the answer sheet other than with the answers you choose. The answer sheet probably will be scanned by a computer, and stray marks will result in a wrong answer being recorded.

Proceed through the whole test answering those questions that you know, or are fairly certain of, the answer. When you have completed these questions, return to those that created doubt when you first read them, categorizing them as suggested previously. Allocate time to each of these depending on the length of time yet available. In answering the questions, think about related clinical situations or basic principles of nursing or sciences being tested or applied in the question. This may help you decide on the correct answer.

In multiple-choice questions, there is a stem and there are several options. In this book there are four options for each question. Only one option is the intended correct answer.

The stem states the question being asked. Read the stem carefully; it will give you direction as to the intended correct answer. As stated previously, many knowledgeable persons do not score well on examinations because they do not read the instructions or the question itself. Some experienced persons also read into the question more than what was intended. Others get frustrated if no option contains the answer they would choose. The best advice is to choose the *best* of the four options even if, in a similar situation, you might do something else that is not mentioned.

If you are not certain about the correct answer to the situation posed by the question, start by eliminating options that you know are not correct. You probably can eliminate two of the four that way. Choosing between the remaining two gives you a 50% probability of answering correctly.

This raises the question of whether or not to guess. If there is a correction for guessing in the examination, the directions on the test must state that fact. A correction for guessing means that the examiners will use a formula to deduct a certain percentage of wrong answers from correct answers for a final score. If there is a correction for guessing *and* you can narrow down the four options to two possible ones, guess; otherwise, do not guess. If there is not a correction for guessing, then guess. Usually test writers and developers use a random assignment of answers to questions. That means there is no pattern of so many 1s, 2s, 3s, and 4s. So if you are guessing, do not worry about the pattern of numbers in the responses that occur in prior or subsequent questions. If you have no knowledge about the correct answer and intend to guess one option, it is also generally safer to select the first or second option.

One last comment about guessing: Some people reject the idea of guessing because, in their opinion, it connotes a behavioral characteristic that is not appropriate in nursing. Test-taking behaviors are not the same as nursing behaviors. There is no evidence to support the supposition that a nurse who guesses on an examination will also guess in deciding about appropriate patient care.

Another point in test taking is the question of changing your answer. Many test-taking advisors recommend that you do not change your answer because the first response you select is generally the correct one. Research on this subject in the past few years reveals a conflicting opinion: Subjects who changed answers did better than those who did not, but this was only when the person taking the test was able to reconsider the response and thought it better to choose a different answer— perhaps other questions in the examination triggered data or knowledge about a previous question that was not considered initially. Therefore, if you believe you have reconsidered sufficiently and

wish to change the answer, do so. Remember to erase completely so that it will not appear that you have a double set of answers on the answer sheet.

After the Examination

The examination is completed. You leave the test site and meet your colleagues who also took the examination. It would be contrary to human nature to suppose that you will not discuss the test and specific questions, but know that doing so may increase your stress level unnecessarily. Your opinion about a correct answer is just as valid as the next person's opinion. Arguing about it or feeling that you selected the wrong option is counterproductive. The questions you remember are most likely the ones you had to devote time in considering the correct option; there were many more that you answered with ease and confidence. Scoring of the examination is based on the total number of questions. Do not let concern about a few questions cause you undue stress.

Another factor after the examination is the sharing of specific questions on the examination with others who have not taken the examination and who wish to review content areas. Some testing bodies attempt to prohibit this; others state that this is not a problem because different questions are used for each test administration. In general, certification examinations are given to evaluate whether a person has the knowledge, skill, and ability to perform specific specialist functions. There are review mechanisms available for all who wish to become certified. Unusual help or specific sharing of questions, where this is deemed to be a problem by the certifying body, casts doubt about the integrity of the entire process.

Unfortunately the ability to use the test as a learning tool is not usually possible, but the review process and the opportunity to test your knowledge contribute to your continued learning and to your practice as a specialist.

2
Standards of Practice and Education

Deborah L. Volker, Mary Cunningham, Judith L. Johnson, and Mary B. Johnson

Select the BEST answer for all of the following questions:

1. The *ANA/ONS Standards of Oncology Nursing Practice* can be used to
   A. develop a conceptual framework for cancer nursing education programs.
   B. assist in the development of performance-evaluation tools.
   C. develop institution-specific patient care standards.
   D. all of the above.

2. The **Professional Development** standard from the *ANA/ONS Standards of Oncology Nursing Practice* states that "the oncology nurse assumes responsibility for professional development and continuing education and contributes to the professional growth of others." Process criteria of this standard include all of the following **EXCEPT**
   A. maintains an awareness of personal beliefs and value systems and their effect on client care.
   B. adheres to policy and procedures.
   C. continually updates his or her knowledge on political, cultural, social, and ethical issues related to oncology.
   D. collaborates with the multidisciplinary team in establishing outcomes for clients.

3. The oncology nurse is expected to implement care to achieve the identified patient outcomes. Which of the following is an example of a *structure* criterion that indicates this standard was met?
   A. Nursing interventions are documented in a timely manner.
   B. Nursing-care plans reflect individualized interventions.
   C. The oncology nurse implements nursing interventions in a caring manner.
   D. Interventions are revised based on the patient's clinical status.

4. The oncology nurse contributes to the scientific base of nursing practice and the field of oncology through the review and application of research. Which of the following statements reflects an *outcome* criterion that indicates this standard was met?
   A. Patient care problems are identified and addressed through research projects.
   B. Agency policy is supportive of research in oncology nursing.
   C. The oncology nurse identifies researchable problems related to practice.
   D. Oncology nurses are provided resource materials regarding research in oncology nursing.

1. *Answer:* **D**

   Rationale: The standards define the scope of cancer nursing practice and, as such, should form the basis for oncology nursing programs, including clinical practice, education, administration, and research.

2. *Answer:* **D**

   Rationale: Statement D is a process criterion of the **Multidisciplinary Collaboration** standard from *ANA/ONS Standards of Oncology Nursing Practice*.

3. *Answer:* **B**

   Rationale: A structure criterion describes resources, people, equipment, or facilities necessary for achievement of the standard. Response B refers to a resource. Responses A and D are outcome criteria. Response C is a process criterion.

4. *Answer:* **A**

   Rationale: An outcome criterion describes the end result of compliance with the standard. Response A is an outcome statement. Responses B and D are structure criteria. Response C is a process criterion.

5. The 11 high-incidence problem areas in oncology nursing cited in the *ANA/ONS Standards of Oncology Nursing Practice* are
   A. key areas where oncology nurses assess, plan, and intervene.
   B. problems that most often impact the patient in the acute care setting.
   C. clinical indicators that are measurable dimensions of the quality of patient care.
   D. the problems with the highest incidence rates.

6. A method to ensure continued professional competency is
   A. peer review.
   B. a quality-assurance audit.
   C. a time and motion study.
   D. a standards review.

7. The following are descriptions of certification. Select the **INCORRECT** statement.
   A. Certification is a process by which a nongovernmental agency grants recognition to individuals who attain a specified level of knowledge and skill in an area of practice.
   B. The primary objective of certification is to protect the certified individual by acknowledging competency to practice and fulfillment of minimal standards.
   C. Certification is one measure of continued competency and a means of documenting, to some extent, continued professional development.
   D. Through the certification process, a specialty nursing association contributes to the establishment of nursing as a profession.

8. An intended outcome of the *ONS Standards of Oncology Education: Patient/Family and Public* is to
   A. delineate strategies for teaching tool development.
   B. improve consistency and accuracy of information included in patient teaching.

   C. improve health promotion and care for the public.
   D. provide guidelines for content.

9. In order to promote effective patient education, resources must be adequate to achieve the learning objectives. Which of the following criteria demonstrates achievement of this standard?
   A. Teaching sessions are based on identified learning needs.
   B. Printed teaching tools are available in the patient's primary language.
   C. Content taught includes community resources available for cancer care.
   D. The patient and family are able to demonstrate psychomotor skills required for self-care.

10. Of the following statements, identify one that is **NOT** a rationale for providing structured patient education.
   A. The adaptation process is enhanced by patient education.
   B. Patient education is a means for providing options and facilitating self-care.
   C. Information is made available in a consistent manner.
   D. Patient education ensures that the patient will be compliant with treatment.

11. In developing an education program for patients who have completed their first regimen of chemotherapy, you need to develop a set of objectives or expected outcomes. Which of the following objectives would be difficult to measure? Upon completion of this educational program the patient will be able to
   A. describe strategies for managing common side effects of chemotherapy.
   B. understand the role of chemotherapy in cancer treatment.
   C. identify community resources available for cancer care.
   D. state side effects that must be reported.

5.   *Answer:* **A**

   Rationale: The 11 high-incidence areas refer to clinical problems that oncology patients most often experience, regardless of the care setting.

6.   *Answer:* **A**

   Rationale: Peer review is a measure of professional competency.

7.   *Answer:* **B**

   Rationale: The primary objective is to protect the consumer by identifying those competent to practice by acknowledging the nurse's additional knowledge and expertise within a specialty beyond licensure requirements.

8.   *Answer:* **C**

   Rationale: The *Standards* provide guidelines for the development, implementation, and evaluation of patient-teaching and public-education programs.

9.   *Answer:* **B**

   Rationale: Response B is the only choice that describes a resource. Teaching tools are most effective when available in the patient's primary language. Response C refers to curricular content; response D, the learners' outcome; and response A, the teaching–learning process.

10.   *Answer:* **D**

   Rationale: When patient education provides options and choices, it promotes patients making informed decisions as partners in their health care. This self-care model may or may not lead to compliance. For example, as an informed decision-maker, the patient may choose not to be treated.

11.   *Answer:* **B**

   Rationale: A well-stated objective identifies a behavior or an action that can be measured.

12. Personal behaviors and public policy related to cancer prevention, detection, control, rehabilitation, and supportive care are influenced by formal and informal cancer public education. Which of the following indicates achievement of this standard?

    A. Public education programs include signs and symptoms of common cancers.

    B. Maintenance of an environment conducive to learning.

    C. The oncology nurse provides leadership in the development of public education materials.

    D. The public reached by cancer education participates in cancer-screening activities.

13. Participation in cancer-related public education is an important nursing activity because

    A. these programs have potential impact on cancer prevention, incidence, morbidity, and mortality.

    B. these programs enhance the professional image of cancer nursing.

    C. participation will modify participants' health behaviors.

    D. the competency of the nurse as a cancer-patient educator will improve.

14. Which of the following statements is **NOT** a learning principle?

    A. Life experiences influence learning.

    B. People will learn when they feel a need to learn.

    C. Learning needs to be reinforced.

    D. Learning is maximized when it is subject-centered.

15. Prior to teaching a patient about prevention and early detection of colorectal cancer, the nurse should

    A. help the patient identify personal risk factors for colorectal cancer.

    B. discuss the need to comply with screening activities.

    C. evaluate the patient's readiness to learn.

    D. assess the patient's normal bowel patterns.

16. Selection of appropriate teaching tools that reflect patient attributes, such as age, culture, and cognitive ability, is best facilitated by

    A. reviewing the literature for available tools.

    B. conducting a learning needs assessment.

    C. determining the cost of available tools.

    D. identifying support services in the home setting.

17. A 48-year-old woman is admitted to the oncology unit following a lumpectomy for a malignant breast tumor. Once her incision heals, she is to have radiation therapy. Which of the following depicts the most appropriate nursing diagnosis category and etiology for this woman during her hospital stay?

    A. Active Role in Health Maintenance r/t Surgery (Mastectomy).

    B. Knowledge Deficit r/t Mastectomy.

    C. Anxiety r/t Knowledge Deficit of Breast Cancer and Treatment.

    D. Alteration in Comfort r/t Breast Cancer and Mastectomy.

18. An effective way by which mass media reaches the public with education about the need for a healthy lifestyle as a way of decreasing the likelihood of cancer is

    A. inappropriate language and settings.

    B. unrealistic suggestions for health maintenance.

    C. failure to dispel myths regarding cancer.

    D. use of celebrities as role models.

19. Nursing interventions that assist the client to overcome a knowledge deficit regarding cancer include all of the following **EXCEPT**

    A. use of external motivators to stimulate learning.

    B. provision of adequate time for learning.

    C. writing materials at the appropriate level.

    D. requesting return demonstration of skills such as breast self-exam.

12. *Answer:* **D**

Rationale: According to the *ONS Standards,* the public reached by cancer education will participate in screening activities.

13. *Answer:* **A**

Rationale: Participation in public cancer-related programs is believed to positively impact cancer prevention and detection activities and, ultimately, cancer morbidity and mortality.

14. *Answer:* **D**

Rationale: Adults are more motivated to learn when learning is problem-centered rather than subject-centered. Problem solving is a kind of learning that creates active participation on the part of the learner.

15. *Answer:* **C**

Rationale: Teaching–learning theories dictate that effective teaching is based on an assessment of the patient's readiness to learn, learning needs, and situational and psychosocial factors that influence learning.

16. *Answer:* **B**

Rationale: A learning needs assessment will identify the patient characteristics that guide selection of teaching materials that are best suited to the individual.

17. *Answer:* **C**

Rationale: Etiologies consist of behaviors of the client, factors in the environment, or an interaction of both. A medical diagnosis is not considered appropriate because it does not individualize the cause of the problem. Knowledge deficit is most appropriately used as an etiology in this case because it probably is an influencing factor of the anxiety.

18. *Answer:* **D**

Rationale: In actuality, the use of well-known and/or easily recognized persons to talk about cancer prevention is effective, as shown by a review of successful mass media education (e.g., the Great American Smokeout).

19. *Answer:* **A**

Rationale: The use of external motivators alone may result in the client learning to please the teacher rather than learning in order to cope more effectively with the various aspects of cancer.

REFERENCES

American Nurses' Association (1976). *Guidelines for Review of Nursing Care at the Local Level.* Kansas City: American Nurses' Association.

American Nurses' Association (1980). *Nursing: A Social Policy Statement.* Kansas City: American Nurses' Association.

American Nurses' Association and Oncology Nursing Society (1987). *Standards of Oncology Nursing Practice.* Kansas City: American Nurses' Association.

Baggs J, Schmitt M, (1988). Collaboration Between Nurses and Physicians. *Image* 20 (3): 145–149.

Challela M, (1979). The Interdisciplinary Team: A Role Definition for Nursing. *Image* 11 (1): 9–16.

Fernsler JI, (1991). Developing Strategies for Public Education in Cancer, in, Baird SB, McCorkle R, Grant M (eds). *Cancer Nursing: A Comprehensive Textbook,* Philadelphia: W B Saunders, pp. 932–943.

Gunning C, (1983). The Profession Itself as A Source of Stress, in, Jacobson S, McGrath H, (eds). *Nurses Under Stress.* New York: John Wiley and Sons, pp. 113–126.

Longman AJ, (1990). Cancer Nursing Education, in, Groenwald SL, Frogge MH, Goodman M, Yarbro CH (eds). *Cancer Nursing: Principles and Practice,* (2nd ed). Boston: Jones and Bartlett, pp. 1256–1269.

Kilman R, Thomas K, (1977). Developing a Forced-choice Measure of Conflict-handling Behavior: The MODE Instrument. *Educational and Psychological Measurement.* 37 (4): 309–325.

Johnson JL, Johnson M, (1992). Dissemination of Information Through Patient and Public Education, in, Clark JC, McGee RF, (eds). *Core Curriculum for Oncology Nursing,* (2nd ed). Philadelphia: W B Saunders.

Marker C, (1987). The Marker Model: A Hierarchy for Nursing Standards. *Journal of Nursing Quality Assurance.* 1 (2): 9–20.

Miaskowski C, Rostad M, (1990). Implementing the ANA/ONS Standards of Oncology Nursing Practice. *Journal of Nursing Quality Assurance.* 4 (3): 15–23.

Morra M, (1991). Developing Strategies for Patient Education in Cancer, in, Baird SB, McCorkle R, Grant M (eds). *Cancer Nursing: A Comprehensive Textbook.* Philadelphia: W B Saunders, pp. 944–956.

Paice JA, Donovan MI, (1991). Issues and Strategies in Professional Education, in, Baird SB, McCorkle R, Grant M (eds). *Cancer Nursing: A Comprehensive Textbook.* Philadelphia: W B Saunders, pp. 965–973.

Prescott P, Bowen S, (1985). Physician – Nurse Relationship. *Annals of Internal Medicine.* 37 (4): 309–325.

Yasko JM, (1991). Role Implementation in Cancer Nursing, in, Baird SB, McCorkle R, Grant M (eds). *Cancer Nursing: A Comprehensive Textbook,* Philadelphia: W B Saunders, pp. 21–29.

Volker DL, (1992). Standards of Oncology Nursing Practice, in, Clark JC, McGee RF, (eds). *Core Curriculum for Oncology Nursing,* (2nd ed). Philadelphia: W B Saunders.

Volker DL, (1992). Standards of Oncology Education: Patient, Family and Public, in, Clark JC, McGee RF, (eds). *Core Curriculum for Oncology Nursing,* (2nd ed). Philadelphia: W B Saunders.

3
Cancer Prevention and Detection

Marilyn Frank-Stromborg and Marilyn Davis

Select the BEST answer for all of the following questions:

1. Your hospital has funded the nursing-education department to offer community-based smoking-cessation classes. Which of the following communities would it be most appropriate to target for the classes?
   A. The upper-middle-class community on the north side of town. Individuals in this area are primarily Caucasian.
   B. The east side of town where most of the light industry is located. The industry is primarily white-collar work.
   C. The west side of town that is primarily middle class. Individuals living in this area are a mix of African American and Caucasian.
   D. The south side of town where the majority of economically disadvantaged individuals live. This area is mostly African Americans.

2. Appropriate nursing interventions for facilitating the participation of the elderly in screening and early diagnosis of cancer include all of the following **EXCEPT**
   A. teaching the value of early diagnosis.
   B. reprimanding the elderly who are noncompliant.
   C. encouraging responsibility for self-care.
   D. suggesting the use of assertive techniques.

3. Among the elderly, the factors that preclude their seeking screening and early diagnosis of cancer include all of the following **EXCEPT**
   A. taking aches and pains for granted.
   B. regarding ill health as inevitable.
   C. weaker lay-referral systems.
   D. misleading health information.

4. The goals of working with the poor as individuals or groups include all of the following **EXCEPT**
   A. appropriate use of community resources.
   B. self-management of such issues as nutrition.
   C. reliance on health-care providers as problem solvers.
   D. use of effective coping strategies.

5. Excessive alcohol consumption has **NOT** been associated with which type of cancer?
   A. Buccal cavity.
   B. Large bowel.
   C. Breast.
   D. Gall bladder.

1. *Answer:* **D**

   Rationale: Smoking has increased in those individuals who are blue-collar workers, minority, and economically disadvantaged. The tobacco industry has targeted a great deal of its resources to minority and poor communities. Nurses need to know which *communities* are at high risk for smoking.

2. *Answer:* **B**

   Rationale: Stimulating guilt or hostility in the elderly (or any other age-group for that matter) does not result in learning (change in behavior).

3. *Answer:* **D**

   Rationale: Health information is actually quite specific regarding the value of screening and early diagnosis of cancer in the elderly; the problem may be access to the information.

4. *Answer:* **C**

   Rationale: Reliance on health-care providers prevents the individual or group from developing general problem-solving skills.

5. *Answer:* **D**

   Rationale: Alcohol is a lifestyle risk factor. Many cancer sites can be affected by excessive alcohol intake.

6. The Year 2000 Dietary Objectives of the NCI include all the following **EXCEPT**
- A. decreasing daily consumption of fat from 40% to 25% of total calories.
- B. minimizing consumption of foods preserved by salt-curing.
- C. increasing daily consumption of vitamins A, C, and E.
- D. increasing consumption of fiber from grains, fruits, and vegetables to 20–30 g per day.

7. When working with Mrs. H's family in the waiting room of the oncology unit, you notice that several of the family members smoke. When you mention the hazards of smoking, the following comments are made: "Our grandfather smoked all his life and lived to 90." "There are more dangers breathing the polluted air in this city than smoking." "Every time I try and quit smoking I gain weight." The most appropriate action for the nurse to take at this time is to
- A. launch into a discussion of what constitutes risk factors.
- B. refer the family members to a smoking-cessation program in the community.
- C. explore the relationship between smoking and lung cancer and clarify misconceptions.
- D. explain about the dangers of second-hand smoke to other members of the family.

8. Colon cancer–prevention strategies include which one of the following?
- A. Reduction of red meat in the diet.
- B. Modification of dietary fat intake.
- C. Pursuit of a diet rich in vegetables.
- D. Pursuit of a diet rich in fiber and vegetables.

9. Psychological factors that may contribute to one's likelihood of developing cancer, as well as not coping effectively with it, include all of the following **EXCEPT**
- A. active involvement in self-care.
- B. type A personality.
- C. inability to express hostile feelings.
- D. lack of a close relationship.

10. Of all the risk factors that have been associated with the development of cancer, which one of the following is currently believed to be responsible for the greatest number of cancers?
- A. Occupational exposures.
- B. Personal habits or lifestyles.
- C. Environmental exposures.
- D. Congenital and genetic disorders.

11. Obesity has been named as a risk factor for which of the following cancers?
- A. Stomach cancer.
- B. Breast cancer.
- C. Prostate cancer.
- D. Corpus uteri cancer.

12. In the outpatient setting, you see Mrs. H and obtain a history of the following: she smoked one pack a day for 20 years, does not practice breast self-exam regularly, is a heavy coffee drinker, is infected with condyloma acuminatum (HPV), and follows a diet that is high in fat and low in fiber and fruits and vegetables. Which one of the following risk factors has been clinically proven to be a direct cause of cancer?
- A. A diet high in fat and low in fiber and fruits and vegetables.
- B. Smoking cigarettes.
- C. Coffee consumption.
- D. Infection with HPV.

13. A triad of risk factors for endometrial cancer is
- A. nulliparity, radiation to pelvic area, and Plummer-Vinson syndrome.
- B. obesity, hypertension and diabetes mellitus.
- C. Bowen's disease, nulliparity, and long-term use of conjugated estrogens.
- D. higher socioeconomic class, cancer of the breast, and history of menstrual irregularities.

14. Cryptorchidism puts a child at risk for which one of the following cancers?
- A. Leukemia.
- B. Testicular cancer.
- C. Sarcoma.
- D. Wilm's tumor.

6. *Answer:* **C**

    Rationale: The Year 2000 Goals for the nation are to decrease the mortality of cancer by 50%. These goals require health-care professionals to participate in educating the public. Increasing vitamins is not one of these recommendations. Rather, vitamins can be increased by eating more vegetables and fruits. Diet is a lifestyle risk factor.

7. *Answer:* **C**

    Rationale: Points out the need to explore with patients/family their perceptions of what constitutes risk factors before doing any health teaching. Smoking is a lifestyle risk factor.

8. *Answer:* **D**

    Rationale: A diet high in fiber and vegetables promotes regular excretion of stool.

9. *Answer:* **A**

    Rationale: It has been observed that persons who wish to be educated about their diagnosis and treatment options, as well as be actively involved in decisions, seem to cope more effectively with the disease and to survive longer.

10. *Answer:* **B**

    Rationale: Lifestyle factors are responsible for the greatest number of cancers and are the most amenable to change.

11. *Answer:* **D**

    Rationale: Obesity is a lifestyle risk factor that is significant in corpus uteri cancer.

12. *Answer:* **D**

    Rationale: HPV is a virus that has been directly linked with cervical dysplasia and carcinoma of the cervix. Sexual activity is a lifestyle risk factor.

13. *Answer:* **B**

    Rationale: Endometrial cancer is one of the leading cancers in older women. There is a definite triad of symptoms associated with this cancer. These are personal risk factors.

14. *Answer:* **B**

    Rationale: Cryptorchidism is a personal risk factor that places the child at increased risk for testicular cancer.

15. Which of the following is **NOT** considered a premalignant condition?
    A. Leukoplakia of the mouth.
    B. Dysplasia of the cervix.
    C. Erythroplakia of the mouth.
    D. Crohn's disease.

16. An example of an iatrogenic cancer is
    A. vaginal cancer in the daughter from DES her mother took during pregnancy.
    B. angiosarcoma of the liver from occupational exposure to vinyl chloride.
    C. oral cancer from chewing betel nuts.
    D. lung cancer from exposure to asbestos in the occupational setting.

17. Individuals who have had an organ transplant are at increased risk for cancer. Which cancer occurs most commonly in transplant patients?
    A. Leukemia.
    B. Hodgkin's disease.
    C. Multiple myeloma.
    D. Non-Hodgkin's lymphoma.

18. Of all the classes of chemotherapy given, which class has the strongest potential for carcinogenic activity?
    A. Alkylating agents.
    B. Antimetabolites.
    C. Plant alkaloids.
    D. Antibiotics.

19. Screening recommendations for cervical cancer include
    A. baseline and annual human choriogonadotropin levels.
    B. annual clinical examination beginning at onset of menarche.
    C. Papanicolaou (Pap) smear every one to three years over the age of 20 or with onset of sexual activity.
    D. Pap smear at the time of any evidence of sexually transmitted disease.

20. Which of the following clinical scenarios illustrates primary prevention of cancer?
    A. A school nurse designs a creative program to encourage teenagers to delay sexual activity as well as practice "safe sex."
    B. A public-health nurse receives a grant to purchase a mobile van that will serve low-income housing areas and offer free Pap smears.
    C. An occupational nurse sets up a breast self-exam training program for the women in a factory.
    D. A geriatric nurse-practitioner receives funds from the Association of Retired Persons to distribute Hemoccult® slides to residents of a retirement community.

21. Endpoints for cancer-control prevention and early detection clinical trials may differ from traditional therapeutic trials by
    A. adherence to progression-free and survival endpoints.
    B. developing performance status criteria.
    C. including a measure of quality of life.
    D. encouraging alternative therapies.

22. The American Cancer Society does **NOT** recommend screening for which one of the following cancers?
    A. Lung cancer.
    B. Cervical cancer.
    C. Oral cancer.
    D. Colorectal cancer.

23. Which one of the following screening practices has been shown to be effective in reducing cancer mortality?
    A. Yearly chest x-rays and sputum cytology for lung cancer.
    B. Monthly breast self-exam.
    C. Pap smears at least once every three years for women aged 20 to 70.
    D. Monthly testicular self-examination.

15.   *Answer:* **D**

Rationale: Premalignant conditions predispose the individual to development of cancer. All choices except D are classified as premalignant conditions that are personal risk factors.

16.   *Answer:* **A**

Rationale: DES is a classic example of an iatrogenic cancer.

17.   *Answer:* **D**

Rationale: This is an example of an iatrogenic risk factor. Patients are at increased risk of cancer due to medical treatments.

18.   *Answer:* **A**

Rationale: Alkylating agents have the greatest potential for development of a second malignancy. This is an example of an iatrogenic carcinogen. It is important for nurses to recognize patients that are at increased risk for cancer due to medical treatments.

19.   *Answer:* **C**

Rationale: The American Cancer Society's screening guidelines recommend a Pap smear every three years, after two negative tests one year apart, in women over the age of 20 and in women younger than 20 who are sexually active.

20.   *Answer:* **A**

Rationale: The question requires that the nurse differentiate between primary and secondary prevention of cancer. Responses B, C, and D are examples of screening/detection programs.

21.   *Answer:* **C**

Rationale: Quality of life may be designated as an alternative endpoint in protocols that have equal treatment effects but differ in toxicity.

22.   *Answer:* **A**

Rationale: There are no recommended screening tests for the early detection of lung cancer because it has not been shown to make a difference in mortality from this disease. Since lung cancer is the leading cause of death from cancer, nurses need to understand primary prevention is of utmost importance in lowering the number of lung cancer deaths.

23.   *Answer:* **C**

Rationale: BSE, TSE, and screening for lung cancer have not been shown to reduce cancer mortality. While nurses do advocate BSE and TSE, they need to be aware that research has not shown these self-examination practices to reduce cancer mortality. Early detection may influence survival time.

24. The American Cancer Society recommends that an asymptomatic person **NOT** at high risk for colorectal cancer have which one of the following?
   A. Periodic colonoscopy (every three years) beginning in the third decade of life.
   B. Annual flexible sigmoidoscopy beginning at age 40.
   C. Sigmoidoscopy, beginning at age 50, to be repeated every three to five years after two consecutive annual normal examinations.
   D. Yearly fecal occult blood testing and periodic flexible sigmoidoscopy, beginning at age 40.

25. A screening test with high sensitivity yields
   A. few false negatives.
   B. many false negatives.
   C. few false positives.
   D. many false positives.

26. Prostatic specific antigen (PSA) levels provide data for
   A. screening.
   B. normal prostatic tissue growth.
   C. disease recurrence.
   D. diagnosis.

27. Colorectal screening recommendations do **NOT** include
   A. fecal occult blood testing over the age of 50.
   B. sigmoidoscopy over the age of 50.
   C. fecal occult blood testing for fiber intolerance.
   D. periodic colonoscopy for familial polyposis coli history.

24. *Answer:* **C**

Rationale: The ACS has recommendations for screening asymptomatic individuals who are not at high risk for colorectal cancer, and nurses need to be aware of these in order to educate the general public.

25. *Answer:* **A**

Rationale: The sensitivity of a test is expressed as the fraction

$$\frac{\text{True Positives}}{\text{True Positives + False Negatives}}$$

The fewer false negatives, the more sensitive the test. A test with 100% sensitivity will always be positive in the presence of the disease it tests.

26. *Answer:* **C**

Rationale: Prostatic specific antigen (PSA) is a biochemical marker for prostate cancer. PSA levels are used to follow disease progression.

27. *Answer:* **C**

Rationale: Responses A and B correspond with the American Cancer Society's guidelines for the asymptomatic population. Familial polyposis of the colon is an inherited autosomal dominant trait and is a personal risk factor for colon cancer. People with a family history of this disease should be followed closely for its development. Response C is a nonexistent test.

REFERENCES

The American Cancer Society Recommendations for Periodic Screening Tests, (1989). Atlanta, GA: American Cancer Society.

Belcher A, (1992). Factors Affecting Responses to the Risk for or Actual Diagnosis of Cancer, in, Clark JC, McGee RF (eds). *Core Curriculum for Oncology Nursing,* (2nd ed). Philadelphia: W B Saunders.

Cohen R, Frank-Stromborg M, (1990). Cancer Risk and Assessment, in, Groenwald SL, Frogge MH, Goodman M, Yarbro CH, (eds). *Cancer Nursing Principles and Practice,* (2nd ed). Boston: Jones and Bartlett, pp. 103–118.

Crawley M, (1992). Primary Prevention in Oncology Nursing Practice, in, Clark JC, McGee RF, (eds). *Core Curriculum for Oncology Nursing,* (2nd ed). Philadelphia: W B Saunders.

Davis M, (1992). Secondary Prevention in Oncology Nursing, in, Clark JC, McGee RF, (eds). *Core Curriculum for Oncology Nursing,* (2nd ed). Philadelphia: W B Saunders.

Frank-Stromborg M, (1984). Psychological Impact of the "Cancer" Diagnosis. *Oncology Nursing Forum.* 11 (3): 16–22.

Frank-Stromborg M, (1991). Evaluating Cancer Risk, in, Baird SB, McCorkle R, Grant M, (eds). *Cancer Nursing. A Comprehensive Textbook.* Philadelphia: WB Saunders, pp. 155–189.

McNally JC, Somerville CT, Measkowski C, Rostad M, (eds). (1991). Prevention and Early Detection, in, *Guidelines for Oncology Nursing Practice* (2nd ed). Philadelphia: W B Saunders, pp. 1–54.

Oleske D, Groenwald SL, (1990). Epidemiology of Cancer, in, Groenwald SL, Frogge MH, Goodman M, Yarbro C, (eds). *Cancer Nursing Principles and Practice,* (2nd ed). Boston: Jones and Bartlett, pp. 3–30.

Olsen S, Frank-Stromborg M, (1991). Cancer Screening and Early Detection, in, Baird SB, McCorkle R, Grant M, (eds). *Cancer Nursing. A Comprehensive Textbook.* Philadelphia: WB Saunders, pp. 190–218.

4

Nursing Management of Responses to the Cancer Experience

Jane C. Clark, Rose F. McGee,
and Fredrica A. Preston

Select the BEST answer for each of the following questions:

1. Grief is *defined* as changes in thinking, feeling, and behaving that occur in response to
   A. death of a significant other.
   B. loss of a valued object or person.
   C. disease with an uncertain prognosis.
   D. losses related to the aging process.

2. Which of the following patient responses is **MOST** representative of a dysfunctional grief response?
   A. A 35-year-old post-mastectomy female who, at six weeks after the surgery, avoids hugs and physical contact with family and friends and has not allowed her husband to look at the surgical site.
   B. A 35-year-old widower who prides himself on keeping all of his wife's possessions and visiting her grave daily for the past five years since her death.
   C. A mother who cries continuously and keeps saying, "No, he can't die," as she attends her 21-year-old son who is dying of leukemia.
   D. A 76-year-old male who cared for his wife during the terminal phases of colon cancer and reports nightmares and disturbing dreams one month later.

3. Resolution of the grief process may be facilitated by which of the following interventions?
   A. Encouraging discussion of feelings related to the loss.
   B. Providing sedation as requested or needed.
   C. Restricting visitors to family members only.
   D. Discouraging expression of negative feelings, such as anger.

4. If an individual is admitted to an oncology unit and physical assessment reveals flushing, sweating, jerky hand movements, and asking questions repeatedly, the most probable nursing diagnosis would be which of the following?
   A. Fear.
   B. Phobias.
   C. Low self-esteem.
   D. Anxiety.

1. *Answer:* **B**

    Rationale: All of the responses given may precipitate the grief process, but the best definition of grief is response B.

2. *Answer:* **B**

    Rationale: Response A is more of a body-image problem, which may be a grief response, but is within the normal time limits of adaptive behavioral responses. Responses C and D represent normal grief responses. Response B is the best answer because of the evidence of a prolonged and unresolved grief process.

3. *Answer:* **A**

    Rationale: Responses other than A represent strategies that block grief work and resolution of the loss.

4. *Answer:* **D**

    Rationale: The stem of the question includes the defining characteristics of anxiety. Stimulus is diffuse, thereby ruling out fear. Self-negation, etc., are not included, ruling out response C (low self-esteem).

5. While administering chemotherapy to a young adult female patient, you observe that both she and her husband appear quite anxious. Which of the following responses would be considered an **INAPPROPRIATE** response in dealing with their anxiety?
   A. "I will teach you more about this procedure later, but for now you can observe what I am doing and ask questions as you like."
   B. "You both appear to be quite anxious. Do you have questions or concerns that you want to discuss before we start?"
   C. "You seem to be concerned. Trust me, I have done this hundreds of times. You can both relax, and I will be done in a minute."
   D. "I realize that this experience can be very upsetting. I will tell you about each step of the procedure, and you can keep me informed about your concerns."

6. Antianxiety drugs are not discontinued abruptly because a possible withdrawal effect is
   A. severe depression.
   B. narcolepsy.
   C. seizures.
   D. hypertensive episodes.

7. Mr. L has been placed on an antianxiety drug. He tells you that he feels much calmer but that his mouth is so uncomfortably dry that he is thinking about discontinuing the drug. The most therapeutic response would be to
   A. support him in his decision and hold the daily dose.
   B. assure him that the dry mouth is not as bad as the anxiousness.
   C. explain that the dryness generally diminishes; increase fluid intake.
   D. call the physician and request an order for another antianxiety drug.

8. Which of the following risk factors indicates the highest potential for suicide among depressed individuals?
   A. History of suicide by a close family member.
   B. History of personal threats of suicide.
   C. History of unsuccessful suicide attempts.
   D. History of obsessions with suicidal thoughts.

9. Physical findings most descriptive of a depressed state include
   A. flat affect, lack of spontaneity, minimal eye contact, and slumped posture.
   B. inappropriate affect, disheveled dress, sweaty hands, and tremors.
   C. labile emotions, hyperactivity, sighing respirations, and overtalkativeness.
   D. facial pallor, tense posturing, vocal tremors, and diaphoresis.

10. Which of the following responses by the nurse would be **MOST** therapeutic in helping the patient deal with the somatic complaints often associated with depression?
   A. Validating symptoms and providing prompt treatment or placebos for relief.
   B. Listening nonjudgmentally and trying diversional techniques as a possible method of alleviation.
   C. Explaining that the symptoms are not "real" and, therefore, need no treatment.
   D. Advising the patient to minimize these symptoms, thus conserving energy to fight the disease.

5. *Answer:* **C**

Rationale: Response A represents a therapeutic response in that it is nondemanding, B acknowledges anxiety, and D acknowledges and reassures. Response C negates the feelings of the patient and spouse, which is a nontherapeutic approach.

6. *Answer:* **C**

Rationale: Withdrawal symptoms similar in character to those noted with barbiturates and alcohol have been reported following the abrupt discontinuing of antianxiety drugs.

7. *Answer:* **C**

Rationale: C represents knowledge of the reactions to the drug (generally, side effects diminish, etc.) and a definitive strategy to alleviate. A may lead to symptoms of withdrawal, B negates the feelings of the patient, and D is premature or not indicated.

8. *Answer:* **C**

Rationale: An attempt has more dangerous potential for suicide than personal history or expression of thoughts.

9. *Answer:* **A**

Rationale: Question requires differentiation between presenting symptoms of depression, anxiety, and panic.

10. *Answer:* **B**

Rationale: "Treatment" of somatic aspects of depression is contraindicated because such actions reinforce these maladaptive behaviors and symptoms. To ask the patient to "buck up" is asking the impossible and instilling guilt. The symptoms are "real" to the patient, and diversion may help.

11. Mrs. R is a 76-year-old retired banker who has done well for two years post–pelvic exenteration. Recently she experienced a recurrence. She now has multiple draining fistulae and has been told that she is not a candidate for further treatment. Her son said that her response has been complete withdrawal. She has changed from a meticulous dresser and housekeeper to neglecting both. She refuses to eat, blames herself for not going for regular Pap smears, and depends heavily on diazepam to "get me through the day." She refuses help from her son, saying he is "wasting his time; I deserve to die." Her history reflects developmental, situational, and disease-related characteristics **MOST** suggestive of
    A. role abandonment.
    B. low self-esteem.
    C. neurotic anxiety.
    D. fear of death.

12. An associated nursing diagnosis that is evident for Mrs. R and requires priority in planning and intervention is
    A. self-care deficit.
    B. sleep pattern disturbance.
    C. ineffective family coping: compromised.
    D. potential for injury.

13. Mrs. R was hospitalized for management of the fistulae. Once the drainage was managed effectively, Mrs. R seemed to show more interest in her care. During this phase, the most therapeutic nursing approach to facilitate adaptive behavior would be to
    A. make no demands on Mrs. R for her own care.
    B. transfer responsibility for Mrs. R's care to her family.
    C. positively reinforce Mrs. R's approaches to self-care.
    D. initiate a referral for rehabilitative counseling.

14. The nursing plan included a referral to a patient-to-patient visitation program to assist Mrs. R in adapting to the life changes imposed by the progression of her cancer. Which of the following would provide this service?
    A. Reach to Recovery.
    B. CanSurMount.
    C. National Cancer Institute.
    D. I Can Cope.

15. Which of the following manifestations are most diagnostic of low self-esteem?
    A. Expressions of self-doubt; hesitancy in social situations; fears of rejection.
    B. Expressions of hopelessness, tenseness; feeling of nervousness.
    C. Expressions of loss of control; preoccupation with fears of the future.
    D. Expressions of difficulty in problem solving; irritability; hypervigilance.

16. Fear differs from anxiety with respect to which of the following characteristics?
    A. Specificity of the stimulus.
    B. Potential to be adaptive or maladaptive.
    C. Autonomic nervous system effects.
    D. Associated somatic manifestations.

17. Desensitization is one behavioral treatment used to alleviate identified fears. The goal of desensitization treatment is to
    A. lessen the threat of the feared object through repeated, controlled exposures.
    B. decrease the effects of the stimulus by the use of sensory nerve blocks.
    C. increase resistance to the threat by monitoring physiological responses to exposure.
    D. increase patient control of responses to the stimulus by sensory overload.

11. *Answer:* **B**

Rationale: Self-negation and self-blame are the defining characteristics that differentiate between self-esteem and the other mood states.

12. *Answer:* **D**

Rationale: Diazepam may cause drowsiness, fatigue, and ataxia. These side effects, along with her age and post-surgical status, put her at risk for injury.

13. *Answer:* **C**

Rationale: A represents a therapeutic approach that is nondemanding. B fosters dependency. D is premature, based on the information given. C is a behavioral approach that reinforces the desired behavior and is, therefore, the best response.

14. *Answer:* **B**

Rationale: Reach to Recovery is for mastectomy patients; NCI is for research, referrals, and education; and I Can Cope is educational. CanSurMount is a patient visitation program for all types of cancer.

15. *Answer:* **A**

Rationale: Differentiates between anxiety, grief, etc.

16. *Answer:* **A**

Rationale: Fear is a response to a specific stimulus. Anxiety is induced by a more generalized or unidentified stimulus. Both cause stimulation of the autonomic nervous system, somatic complaints and may be either adaptive or maladaptive.

17. *Answer:* **A**

Rationale: Asks respondent to differentiate between desensitization (A), biofeedback (C) and hypnosis (D).

18. When patients are incapacitated by fears that cancer is "uncontrollable" or by fears of social rejection because of a cancer diagnosis, the nurse should
   A. provide detailed information to dissipate fears.
   B. divert the attention of the patient to avoid discussion.
   C. accept fears as real to facilitate self-expression.
   D. limit patient teaching to the family to spare the patient.

19. In admitting an elderly person with cancer whose physical and psychosocial evaluation reflects a fearful state bordering on panic, the most therapeutic approach is to be
   A. supportive and direct, using soothing voice tones.
   B. authoritative and decisive, enunciating clearly.
   C. thorough and informative, validating knowledge.
   D. detached and objective, minimizing patient fears.

20. The predominant fear for an 18-year-old female with a diagnosis of sarcoma of the tibia to be treated with amputation is
   A. hospitalization.
   B. disfigurement.
   C. desertion.
   D. loss of status.

21. Ms. J is preparing to go home after being hospitalized for cancer therapy. She has had difficulty sleeping in the hospital. Which of the following statements, if made by Ms. J, would indicate a need for additional teaching?
   A. "I will plan to take my pain medicine about thirty minutes before I go to bed."
   B. "I will be able to take my bath just before I go to bed once I get home."
   C. "I will drink just a small glass of warm milk before I go to bed."
   D. "I will plan to take my cortisone about thirty minutes before I go to bed."

22. A 74-year-old patient with lung cancer has had difficulty going to sleep for the past two weeks secondary to shortness of breath. Which of the following screening questions would be **MOST** important in evaluating the impact of his difficulty in going to sleep?
   A. How long are you able to sleep at night?
   B. How rested do you feel on awakening?
   C. How many naps do you take during the day?
   D. How do you help yourself go to sleep?

23. Mr. W has been in the hospital for one week. He is complaining of insomnia. Which of the following signs and symptoms would you expect to see in Mr. W?
   A. Restlessness during the day.
   B. Focused concentration.
   C. Improved problem solving.
   D. Inability to sleep during the day.

24. Mr. J has had difficulty sleeping in the hospital. Which of the following nursing actions is **MOST** likely to promote a restful environment for sleep?
   A. Turning off all lights in the room.
   B. Setting the room temperature at seventy degrees.
   C. Talking to Mr. J about his worries.
   D. Asking Mr. J about his bedtime routines.

18. *Answer:* **C**

Rationale: During times of intense fear, patients will not comprehend detailed information (A) and need to discuss and clarify fears (B and D are, therefore, wrong). Acceptance will facilitate self-expression and allow the patient to work through the fears.

19. *Answer:* **A**

Rationale: During times of intense fear, patients benefit most from a supportive environment in which stimuli are limited (e.g., soothing voice, limited information, etc.).

20. *Answer:* **B**

Rationale: Body image is crucial in adolescents.

21. *Answer:* **D**

Rationale: Insomnia is a common side effect of steroid use. The effect is more common when steroids are taken at bedtime rather than in the morning.

22. *Answer:* **B**

Rationale: Although the amount of sleep is an objective measure of insomnia, the impact of insomnia is a subjective evaluation of perceived feeling of being rested by the patient.

23. *Answer:* **A**

Rationale: Hospitalization often results in sleep pattern disturbances and subjective complaints of not feeling rested. Restlessness is a common side effect of sleep pattern disturbance.

24. *Answer:* **D**

Rationale: Sleep hygiene is an individualized process. Patients are most likely to respond to routines used at home versus those imposed by hospitalization.

25. Mr. S becomes very agitated and defensive during your assessment of his stomach pain. When confronted with his behavior, he states, "What's the use of all these questions? We both know it's just the cancer getting worse." You reply,
   A. "You're probably right; I'll just bring you your pain medicine and let you rest."
   B. "Many people with cancer have pain that is not related to their disease, and the pain can easily be taken care of once we know the cause."
   C. "It's probably just constipation from all the narcotics you need for pain; perhaps a laxative will work."
   D. "You must be worried that the pain means your cancer has spread, but that is not always true."

26. A patient has problems describing her pain and is always so vague that the staff feel they are often treating her pain based on their interpretation. Which of the following would help the nurses manage the patient's pain?
   A. Use a numerical scale (e.g., 1 = no pain; 5 = excruciating) to assess pain.
   B. Begin patient on "round-the-clock" pain medication so she will not have the experience of pain.
   C. Continue with current management since nurses' assessments are usually correct.
   D. Begin the patient on a long-acting narcotic with a short-acting narcotic for breakthrough pain.

27. Ms. B is concerned that she is becoming addicted because she requires an increased dosage of her narcotic. You explain to her that
   A. she ought not to worry about addiction because it happens to everyone on narcotics.
   B. medically induced addiction differs from street addiction.
   C. she is right to worry and you will speak to her physician about changing her narcotic.
   D. she is not addicted but is becoming tolerant to her current dosage.

28. Mrs. B cannot understand why her husband wakes up in pain when he seems to sleep through the night. He doesn't even wake up for his pain medicine which he needs every three hours during the day. Your best advice is:
   A. if he is sleeping, he obviously is not in pain.
   B. wake him up every three hours to take his pain medicine.
   C. speak to the physician about longer-acting pain relievers.
   D. do not wake him up, but medicate him as soon as he gets up.

29. Which of the following is a preventable side effect of narcotic therapy?
   A. Hallucinations.
   B. Anorexia.
   C. Xerostomia.
   D. Constipation.

30. Which of the following could be used as a coanalgesic drug for nerve pain?
   A. Cimetidine.
   B. Aminotriptyline.
   C. Cyclophosphamide.
   D. Diphenhydramine.

31. A 52-year-old woman with breast cancer complains of itching. Which of the following could increase the severity of her pruritus?
   A. Anticholinergics.
   B. Hypercalcemia.
   C. Antihistamines.
   D. Damp climate.

32. A patient received her first dose of sub.q. interferon yesterday. Today she complains of itching and redness at the injection site. The most probable cause is
   A. allergic reaction to interferon.
   B. infection at injection site.
   C. local tissue response at injection site.
   D. local tissue trauma due to poor technique.

25. *Answer:* **D**

   Rationale: Approximately 30% of pain in cancer patients is not cancer related.

26. *Answer:* **A**

   Rationale: Patients need to describe/quantify their pain as a subjective experience.

27. *Answer:* **D**

   Rationale: Tolerance is the need for more medication; it is not addiction.

28. *Answer:* **C**

   Rationale: Longer-acting narcotics provide the patient with a consistent level of pain relief.

29. *Answer:* **D**

   Rationale: Constipation, a common side effect of narcotic therapy, can be prevented by initiation of a bowel regimen.

30. *Answer:* **B**

   Rationale: Tricyclics are effective analgesics for the burning sensation of nerve pain.

31. *Answer:* **B**

   Rationale: Hypercalcemia leads to release of calcium salts, which cause itching.

32. *Answer:* **C**

   Rationale: Itching is part of the inflammatory response to immunotherapy.

33. Which of the following would be included in your self-care instructions for a patient with pruritus?
    A. Take frequent, warm baths to promote vasodilation.
    B. Use petroleum-based lubricants on your skin.
    C. Avoid cutaneous stimulation at the site of itching.
    D. Use water-based lubricants on your skin.

34. Of the following nursing diagnoses, which holds the greatest relevance for pruritus?
    A. Alteration in hygiene.
    B. Alteration in nutrition.
    C. Alteration in fluid status.
    D. Alteration in protective mechanisms.

35. Standard pharmacologic management of pruritus includes
    A. antihistamines.
    B. aminotryptylline.
    C. low-dose folinic acid.
    D. megestral acetate.

36. Because vasodilation may increase the severity of pruritus, the patient should institute which of the following measures?
    A. Take frequent, warm tub baths.
    B. Maintain a dry environment.
    C. Apply cool compresses to site of pruritus.
    D. Increase fluid intake with warm beverages (e.g. tea, coffee, cocoa, etc.).

37. A common drug used to treat hiccoughs is
    A. amitriptyline HCl (Elavil).
    B. dexamethasone (Decadron).
    C. methylphenidate HCl (Ritalin).
    D. chlorpromazine (Thorazine).

38. Mr. L, an elderly gentleman with esophageal cancer, has had hiccoughs for the past four days. You are concerned about which of the following complications?
    A. Dysphagia.
    B. Nausea.
    C. Aspiration.
    D. Dehydration.

39. Which of the following foods would you give to a patient complaining of dysphagia?
    A. Clear broth.
    B. Turkey sandwich.
    C. Yogurt.
    D. Dry toast.

40. M. R. is concerned about her husband's difficulty in swallowing since his radiation therapy. She calls you for advice about dietary modifications. You advise her to
    A. maintain the current diet but have the patient tilt head back to allow passage of food bolus.
    B. provide soft or semi-soft foods.
    C. provide only high-calorie, high-protein liquids to avoid choking.
    D. keep the patient NPO until dysphagia subsides.

41. Mr. S is two weeks postradiation therapy to a field which included his esophagus. He complains of difficulty swallowing and a feeling that food gets "stuck." Which of the following could affect his dysphagia?
    A. Stomatitis.
    B. Tracheostomy.
    C. Dental caries.
    D. Leukopenia.

42. A referral to which team member would be suggested for management of unresolved swallowing problems?
    A. Respiratory therapist.
    B. Speech therapist.
    C. Physical therapist.
    D. Oral surgeon.

43. Which of the following would **NOT** be an appropriate nursing diagnosis for potential complications of dysphagia?
    A. Alteration in nutritional status.
    B. Alteration in fluid and electrolyte balance.
    C. Alteration in protective mechanisms.
    D. Alteration in safety related to potential for aspiration.

33. *Answer:* **D**

    Rationale: Water-soluble lubricants will promote hydration of the skin.

34. *Answer:* **D**

    Rationale: Cancer patients are at risk for infection when skin integrity is impaired.

35. *Answer:* **A**

    Rationale: Itching is related to the release of histamines.

36. *Answer:* **C**

    Rationale: Cool compresses promote capillary constriction.

37. *Answer:* **D**

    Rationale: One of the indications for the use of Thorazine is the relief of intractable hiccoughs.

38. *Answer:* **C**

    Rationale: A potential complication of hiccoughs is aspiration, especially with esophageal cancer.

39. *Answer:* **C**

    Rationale: Soft or pureed foods are the easiest to swallow and least likely to cause aspiration.

40. *Answer:* **B**

    Rationale: Soft or pureed foods are easier to swallow; liquids have an increased risk of being aspirated. The neck should never be hyperextended; it should be tilted forward if any position change is needed.

41. *Answer:* **A**

    Rationale: Oral stomatitis can lead to swallowing difficulties.

42. *Answer:* **B**

    Rationale: The role of a speech therapist includes assistance with swallowing problems.

43. *Answer:* **C**

    Rationale: Potential complications of dysphagia include fluid and electrolyte imbalance, malnutrition, and aspiration.

44. Mrs. C has been diagnosed with tumor lysis syndrome. Which of the following assessments should the nurse make to detect potentially significant electrolyte imbalances?
   A. Blood pressure, heart rate, and neuromuscular exam.
   B. Respiratory rate, bowel elimination pattern, and speech.
   C. Range of motion, gait, and mental status examination.
   D. Urinary output, sleep–wake patterns, and appetite.

45. Mrs. J has lymphoma. She has had a dramatic response to chemotherapy and is at risk for tumor lysis syndrome. Which of the following findings would cue the nurse to a significant electrolyte imbalance?
   A. Tachycardia.
   B. Constipation.
   C. Hypertension.
   D. Muscle cramps.

46. Mrs. S has breast cancer with metastasis to the bone. She is at risk for hypercalcemia. Which of the following assessments would be the initial change indicating clinical symptoms of hypercalcemia?
   A. Respiratory rate.
   B. Muscle tone.
   C. Mental status.
   D. Urinary output.

47. Mr. K is receiving amphotericin and is at risk for hypokalemia. Which assessment would be most important in clinically detecting hypokalemia?
   A. Blood pressure.
   B. Skin turgor.
   C. Deep tendon reflexes.
   D. Appetite.

48. Mr. K has hypokalemia. In evaluating choices that he made on his dietary menu, which of the following choices would indicate a need for additional dietary teaching?
   A. Bananas.
   B. Potato chips.
   C. Gatorade.
   D. Apples.

49. Mrs. C is being treated with high-volume saline infusions for hypercalcemia ($Ca^{++} = 14.5$). Which of the following nursing interventions would be critical in providing safe care for Mrs. C?
   A. Encourage Mrs. C to ask for help when ambulating to the bathroom.
   B. Measure the urine output after every void.
   C. Assist Mrs. C to a bedside commode every one to two hours.
   D. Clean and dry the perineum after each void.

50. Mr. B, an elderly man with lung cancer, presents to the emergency room with a history of vomiting for five days. Physical exam reveals shallow, slow respirations, irregular pulse, and muscle twitching. He appears disoriented and irritable. Blood gases reveal pH (plasma) = 7.4 and bicarbonate = 29 mEq/L. Mr. B is experiencing which complication of prolonged vomiting?
   A. Metabolic alkalosis.
   B. Metabolic acidosis.
   C. Hypernatremia.
   D. Hypokalemia.

51. Mr. P. is receiving combination antiemetic therapy (metoclopramide, lorazepam, and dexamethasone) as part of his chemotherapy protocol. You enter his room and he complains of not being able to open his mouth. He states, "My jaw feels stuck. It just started." The most likely cause is a reaction to
   A. lorazepam.
   B. dexamethasone.
   C. metoclopramide.
   D. chemotherapy drugs.

52. Which drug would be used to reverse a metoclopramide extrapyramidal reaction?
   A. Diphenhydramine.
   B. Lorazepam.
   C. Decadron.
   D. Prochlorperazine.

44. *Answer:* **A**

   Rationale: With tumor lysis syndrome, potassium is released from the intracellular compartment. Excess amounts of potassium result in hyperkalemia, which leads to irregular heart rate and neuromuscular irritability.

45. *Answer:* **D**

   Rationale: With tumor lysis syndrome, calcium is released from the intracellular compartment and results in hypercalcemia. Signs and symptoms include muscle cramps, flaccid paralysis, weakness, paresthesia, EKG changes, diarrhea, nausea, and bradycardia.

46. *Answer:* **C**

   Rationale: Changes in mental status are some of the *initial changes* seen in patients with hypercalcemia.

47. *Answer:* **C**

   Rationale: Signs and symptoms of hypokalemia include muscle weakness, a decrease in deep tendon reflexes, paresthesias, arrhythmias, mental confusion, lethargy, and apathy.

48. *Answer:* **D**

   Rationale: Potassium rich foods include bananas, oranges, potatoes, nuts, potato chips, fruit juices, broth, colas, and Gatorade.

49. *Answer:* **C**

   Rationale: At this level of hypercalcemia, symptoms would include muscle weakness and confusion. The nurse should encourage use of a bedside commode rather than a bedpan. In addition, transfer techniques to the bedside commode are safer than ambulation to the bathroom.

50. *Answer:* **A**

   Rationale: Metabolic alkalosis occurs when fluid volume is depleted and sodium, chloride, and potassium are lost.

51. *Answer:* **C**

   Rationale: Metoclopramide has been known to cause extrapyramidal reactions when administered parenterally.

52. *Answer:* **A**

   Rationale: Diphenhydramine reverses the effects of extrapyramidal reactions to drugs.

53.   Ms. L timidly informs you that every time she comes to the clinic for chemotherapy she begins to feel nauseated, even before she gets her treatment. She cannot understand why this happens. Your response is:
  A.   "Don't worry about it. It happens to everyone."
  B.   "What you are feeling is anticipatory nausea. It is a conditioned response many people experience with chemotherapy."
  C.   "Try to eat before coming to the clinic. This will decrease that queasy feeling."
  D.   "Do not eat after 12 A.M. the night before your clinic appointment. This will decrease your chance of vomiting."

54.   Mrs. S has just completed an infusion of 120 mg cisplatin. She had an antiemetic protocol of metoclopramide (Reglan), lorazepam (Ativan) and dexamethasone (Decadron). Upon discharge from the clinic she is given a prescription for Torecan. You instruct her as follows:
  A.   "You had enough antiemetics here in the clinic. You will not have any problems at home."
  B.   "Take your antiemetic only if you feel sick."
  C.   "Take your antiemetic every four to six hours around-the-clock for the next two days, then every four hours as needed."
  D.   "Do not eat for the next twenty-four hours to avoid nausea and try to avoid taking more medications."

55.   All of the following interventions help to relieve nausea **EXCEPT**
  A.   medicating with an antiemetic each time vomiting is experienced.
  B.   avoiding fatty or spicy foods.
  C.   medicating with an antiemetic on a round-the-clock basis until nausea subsides.
  D.   using relaxation or visual imagery techniques.

56.   Which of the following drugs has the highest emetogenic potential?
  A.   Cisplatin.
  B.   Vinblastine.
  C.   Etoposide.
  D.   Bleomycin.

57.   Which of the following is **NOT** an important factor to consider in the assessment of taste alterations in persons with cancer?
  A.   Taste alterations can lead to anorexia.
  B.   Taste alterations can lead to positive nitrogen balance.
  C.   Taste alterations can indicate stomatitis.
  D.   Taste alterations can indicate disease progression.

58.   Mrs. B is worried about her husband's nutrition. Since starting chemotherapy, he states, "Nothing tastes right." What advice would you give Mrs. B?
  A.   "Continue to prepare meals as usual. Eventually his taste will return to normal (about two weeks post therapy)."
  B.   "There is nothing you can do; this happens to everyone on chemotherapy."
  C.   "Try to increase his intake of meat, because it is a good source of protein and is generally well tolerated."
  D.   "Try to increase sensitivity of taste buds by using spices and herbs in meal preparation."

59.   Mr. P has completed a course of radiation therapy for head and neck cancer. Which of the following would be an added risk factor for his development of taste changes?
  A.   Steroid therapy.
  B.   Stomatitis.
  C.   Cyclophosphamide therapy.
  D.   Hepatic toxicity.

60.   A common taste alteration is a
  A.   decreased threshold for sweets.
  B.   craving for red meats.
  C.   sweet taste in the mouth.
  D.   decreased threshold for bitter tastes.

53. *Answer:* **B**

Rationale: Psychogenic factors play a role in feelings of nausea.

54. *Answer:* **C**

Rationale: Antiemetics must be taken on a consistent, round-the-clock basis. Some chemotherapy drugs can have emetic potential up to seventy-two hours after treatment.

55. *Answer:* **A**

Rationale: Medicating after vomiting does little to relieve the nausea that preceded the emesis.

56. *Answer:* **A**

Rationale: Cisplatin has a high emetic potential (75%) related to stimulation of the chemoreceptor trigger zone (CTZ).

57. *Answer:* **B**

Rationale: Taste alterations can lead to anorexia, which can lead to negative nitrogen balance.

58. *Answer:* **D**

Rationale: Spices and flavorings can enhance taste sensations altered by chemotherapy.

59. *Answer:* **B**

Rationale: Oral infections can interfere with taste.

60. *Answer:* **D**

Rationale: A decreased threshold for bitter tastes is due to negative nitrogen balance.

61.   In instructing Mr. J about self-care while on radiation therapy, which of the following statements would indicate a need for further teaching?
- A.   "I'm so glad it's the weekend; no RT for two days and I don't have to do all of that mouth care until Monday."
- B.   "I'm going to throw out my Cepacol and start using baking soda and water."
- C.   "So much for my scotch and soda before dinner!"
- D.   "I guess I better get these dentures checked. They've been bothering me since I lost all that weight."

62.   Which would **NOT** be a key assessment factor of a patient with xerostomia?
- A.   Overall status of teeth and gums.
- B.   Impact of xerostomia on daily life.
- C.   Status of mucous membranes.
- D.   Pattern of elimination.

63.   Which of the following nursing diagnoses would most likely be associated with xerostomia?
- A.   Alteration in elimination.
- B.   Alteration in nutrition.
- C.   Alteration in body image.
- D.   Knowledge deficit about treatment outcomes.

64.   A patient, after receiving radiation therapy to the head and neck for one week, complains of difficulty chewing, swallowing and speaking. He has no appetite. His oral mucous membranes are dry, and his saliva is thick and scanty. He denies pain. He most likely has
- A.   stomatitis.
- B.   herpes simplex.
- C.   buccal inflammation.
- D.   xerostomia.

65.   Xerostomia is
- A.   chronic inflammation of the salivary glands.
- B.   dryness of the skin.
- C.   an infection of the oral cavity.
- D.   mouth dryness.

66.   Mr. J is to begin radiation therapy to a field which includes the salivary glands. Which of the following factors would increase his risk for developing xerostomia?
- A.   Alcohol ingestion.
- B.   Digitalis preparations.
- C.   Poor dentation.
- D.   Steroid therapy.

67.   Mrs. P does not worry about her lack of appetite and decreased caloric intake. She has not been as active since starting her chemotherapy and feels she is not expending as many calories. The nurse's advice is:
- A.   "Your appetite will return when your treatment is completed."
- B.   "Your caloric intake demands are increased when on chemotherapy."
- C.   "Try to gain weight because the heavier you are, the greater the dose of chemotherapy you will receive."
- D.   "Weight loss is inevitable for patients on chemotherapy, and you should just try to eat what you can during this time."

68.   Despite a dramatic decrease in appetite and caloric intake, Ms. T's weight has increased by 3 kg and her abdomen and ankles are swollen. Ms. T's lab results related to this would reveal
- A.   hyperkalemia.
- B.   hypoalbuminemia.
- C.   hypomagnecemia.
- D.   hypourecemia.

69.   Mrs. D calls to tell you how upset she is that her husband "doesn't eat like he used to." She fears he will never get better, and mealtimes have become a source of friction. Nursing intervention would include
- A.   informing the patient that he must eat or he will not be eligible for further treatment.
- B.   supporting the wife in her current efforts to force-feed the patient for his benefit.
- C.   placing the patient on supplemental feedings to avoid further marital friction.
- D.   encouraging the wife to provide the patient with more frequent, smaller meals.

61. *Answer:* **A**

    Rationale: The oral care program continues even during a weekend hiatus from radiation therapy.

62. *Answer:* **D**

    Rationale: Xerostomia relates to conditions of the oral cavity.

63. *Answer:* **B**

    Rationale: Xerostomia leads to difficulty in chewing and swallowing foods.

64. *Answer:* **D**

    Rationale: Patients with xerostomia have dry mucous membranes and difficulty with oral intake. Pain is not a factor.

65. *Answer:* **D**

    Rationale: This is the definition of xerostomia.

66. *Answer:* **A**

    Rationale: Alcohol use dries mucous membranes.

67. *Answer:* **B**

    Rationale: While on chemotherapy or radiation therapy, caloric intake requirements increase by two calories per pound.

68. *Answer:* **B**

    Rationale: Decreased protein intake leads to reduced albumin, resulting in third spacing of fluids.

69. *Answer:* **D**

    Rationale: Smaller, more frequent meals are usually tolerated better than fewer, larger ones.

70. A 76-year-old man recently diagnosed with metastatic lung cancer lives alone and has few friends or family around. He complains of "just no appetite anymore." Your assessment reveals a ten-pound weight loss in the past month. Which of the following would be an **INAPPROPRIATE** referral?
   A. Social service for Meals on Wheels.
   B. A cancer support group.
   C. Local church for volunteer services.
   D. Nutrition support team for evaluation of need for parenteral nutrition.

71. Risk factors associated with anorexia include all **EXCEPT**
   A. recent treatment for cancer.
   B. unintentional weight loss of at least 10% within six months.
   C. depression.
   D. living alone.

72. Select the drug(s) from the following list of chemotherapy agents which have the **lowest** potential to cause alopecia.
   A. Doxorubicin and cyclophosphamide.
   B. Methotrexate with leucovorin rescue.
   C. Bolus doses of doxorubicin.
   D. Cyclophosphamide, methotrexate, 5-FU.

73. Which of the following treatments is most likely to cause permanent hair loss?
   A. MOPP therapy for Hodgkin's disease.
   B. 6000 cGy radiation for brain tumor.
   C. CMF for breast cancer.
   D. High-dose ARA-C for leukemia.

74. Prevention of hair loss, inherent with the administration of chemotherapy drugs, by the use of scalp hypothermia and scalp tourniquets is rejected by some oncologists based on the concern that the intervention may
   A. lead to incomplete cell kill.
   B. cause undue discomfort.
   C. lead to a stroke.
   D. cause damage to hair follicles.

75. Patients often question the pattern of hair loss and regrowth with chemotherapy. Select the most accurate estimate of the usual pattern of regrowth.
   A. One to two weeks after completion of chemotherapy.
   B. One to two months after completion of chemotherapy.
   C. Three to four months after completion of chemotherapy.
   D. Five to six months after completion of chemotherapy.

76. Patient teaching for individuals receiving high doses of chemotherapy drugs, known to have a high potential for causing hair loss, should include which of the following suggestions?
   A. Hair loss occurs slowly; therefore, adequate time will be available to make plans once the loss begins to occur.
   B. Hair texture and color will be the same as before any loss occurs; therefore, wigs should closely resemble original hair.
   C. Hair loss is likely; therefore, the best match and the best time psychologically for a wig purchase may be prior to therapy.
   D. Hair appears thicker with a permanent or with a color application; therefore, hair should be permed or colored to lessen evidence of possible hair loss.

77. Which of the following statements is an accurate assessment of the relationship between chemotherapy and alopecia?
   A. Hair loss is generally permanent.
   B. Axillary and pubic hair are spared.
   C. Drug dosage does not affect severity.
   D. Drugs vary in potential for causing hair loss.

70. *Answer:* **D**

Rationale: Parenteral nutrition does not improve appetite in patients with advanced cancer.

71. *Answer:* **B**

Rationale: The cause of anorexia is often multidimensional—physical and psychosocial.

72. *Answer:* **B**

Rationale: Tests application of knowledge that combination therapy (A and D) and route of administration (bolus versus slow infusion) influence hair loss. Responses B and C are both single dose, but the bolus administration would be the differentiating factor.

73. *Answer:* **B**

Rationale: Chemotherapy generally causes temporary hair loss; radiation doses above 4500 cGy generally induce permanent loss. This is important information for patient teaching.

74. *Answer:* **A**

Rationale: Patients with disseminated metastases, scalp metastases, or hematologic malignancies may experience decreased exposure to the chemotherapeutic agent. They may subsequently experience a high rate of metastasis.

75. *Answer:* **B**

Rationale: Regrowth is rare before one month and after six months.

76. *Answer:* **C**

Rationale: Responses A, B, and D contain incorrect information (loss generally is faster with high doses of drugs with high potential for alopecia). Perms and color may damage hair, thus increasing hair loss. The remaining response, C, requires knowledge of hair changes on regrowth and timing of nursing interventions.

77. *Answer:* **D**

Rationale: High doses of chemotherapy cause atrophy of the hair root bulb. Lower doses cause partial atrophy and thinning, rather than the spontaneous loss seen with high-dose therapy. A higher percentage of pubic and axillary hair is in the resting, versus mitotic, stage; therefore, it is spared. Knowledge of the difference in potential of drugs to cause alopecia is important to clarify public misconceptions that all chemotherapy causes alopecia.

78. Mrs. S is receiving chemotherapy for treatment of lymphoma. Diagnostic tests prior to initiation of therapy revealed no evidence of bone marrow involvement. As the nurse caring for Mrs. S, which of the following assessments would be most important in evaluating critical hematologic toxicity from the chemotherapy?
   , A. Bruising of skin.
   B. Strength of muscles.
   C. Degree of fatigue.
   D. Rate of breathing.

79. Mrs. J has a platelet count of 20,000 following chemotherapy for acute leukemia. Which of the following orders, written by a new intern on the service, should be questioned by the nurse caring for Mrs. J?
   A. Acetaminophen 650 mg po q 4 hr for pain.
   B. Stool softener po qd prn for constipation.
   C. Apply direct pressure to all venipuncture sites for five minutes.
   D. May take temperature rectally when patient is using oxygen.

80. A nurse is developing a standard of care for a client experiencing thrombocytopenia. Which of the following routine assessments would be most important in evaluating the risk of bleeding in the client with thrombocytopenia?
   A. Presence of diarrhea.
   B. Presence of constipation.
   C. Presence of fever.
   D. Presence of pus.

81. Mr. G is thrombocytopenic following combination chemotherapy and radiation. Which of the following changes in Mr. G's symptoms may indicate complications of thrombocytopenia?
   A. Tarry stools.
   B. Diarrhea.
   C. Fever.
   D. Urticaria.

82. Mrs. K has been receiving adriamycin and cisplatin therapy for ovarian cancer. Her platelet count is 20,000. Which of the following statements, if made by Mrs. K, would indicate to the nurse the need for additional teaching?
   A. "I will let the nurse know if I notice any blood in my urine."
   B. "My daughter got me an electric toothbrush so that I can perform good mouth care."
   C. "Excessive bruising is one sign that my platelet count is low."
   D. "My husband got me an electric razor so that I could shave my legs safely."

83. Mr. J is experiencing severe thrombocytopenia related to bone marrow invasion from multiple myeloma. Which of the following actions would be most important in providing nursing care for Mr. J?
   A. Teach the patient self-care skills that minimize the risk of trauma (e.g., use a soft toothbrush).
   B. Encourage dietary selections that are high in protein and calories, such as meat, cheese, and eggs.
   C. Apply firm pressure to all venipuncture sites for at least one minute.
   D. Report blurred vision and restlessness immediately.

84. Mr. H received chemotherapy approximately two weeks ago. Laboratory tests results are as follows: WBC = 3000, segs = 15%, bands = 10%, eosinophils = 5%, and lymphs = 60%. Mr. H's absolute granulocyte count is
   A. 450
   B. 750
   C. 900
   D. 1800

85. Which of the following assessments would alert the nurse to an increased risk for infection during chemotherapy treatments?
   A. Age = 36 years.
   B. Well-balanced diet.
   C. Current steroid therapy.
   D. Weight = 160 pounds.

78. *Answer:* **A**

Rationale: Although most chemotherapeutic agents have some degree of marrow toxicity, the cells most likely to be affected are platelets and white blood cells. Answers B, C and D refer to symptomatology commonly seen in clients with anemia. Bruising of the skin would be the most important finding because spontaneous bleeding would be a critical sequela.

79. *Answer:* **D**

Rationale: Invasive procedures, including rectal temperatures, should be avoided when the platelet count is severely decreased.

80. *Answer:* **B**

Rationale: The Valsalva maneuver increases intracranial pressure and increases the risk for intracranial bleeding.

81. *Answer:* **A**

Rationale: Tarry stools are indicative of bleeding from the upper portion of the gastrointestinal tract and/or old blood.

82. *Answer:* **B**

Rationale: An electric toothbrush is too harsh for cleaning debris from the teeth and mouth when the platelet count is 20,000. The oral mucous membranes are traumatized, and bleeding from the gums may occur.

83. *Answer:* **D**

Rationale: Intracranial bleeding in the presence of thrombocytopenia is an emergency situation. Blood occupies a limited-space environment; therefore, the risks of increased intracranial pressure and subsequent tissue damage are present.

84. *Answer:* **B**

Rationale: The absolute granulocyte count (AGC) is determined by the formula AGC = WBC × (% segs + % bands). The absolute granulocyte count provides a measure of the number of mature granulocytes available to fight infection.

85. *Answer:* **C**

Rationale: Steroid therapy decreases the ability of mature granulocytes to move from the vascular compartment into the tissues.

86. Mr. S has completed a ten-day course of chemotherapy for acute leukemia. His family wishes to be involved in his care. Which of the following actions, if taken by a family member, would indicate an understanding of risks associated with immunosuppression?
  A. Taking pictures of Mr. S's dog to hang in his hospital room.
  B. Bringing Mr. S's 4-year-old son to visit each day after kindergarten.
  C. Bringing cut flowers from Mr. S's garden to the hospital.
  D. Having family members come to visit in groups rather than one at a time.

87. Mrs. J is preparing to go home following a course of chemotherapy for acute leukemia. Her white blood count is 1500. Which of the following statements, if made by Mrs. J, would indicate a need for additional teaching?
  A. "I should limit contact with large crowds of people."
  B. "I should call my doctor if I have a fever greater than 101°F."
  C. "I should get my flu shot before I leave the hospital."
  D. "I should continue careful handwashing and mouth care."

88. Mrs. J is being treated for acute leukemia. She received her first course of Cytosar and daunomycin two weeks ago. Which of the following self-care measures would be the most important to teach Mrs. J?
  A. Floss teeth after each meal with unwaxed dental floss.
  B. Avoid washing hair more than once a week.
  C. Wash hands thoroughly after each use of the bathroom.
  D. Exercise caution when shaving legs with a razor.

89. Mr. G is two weeks post chemotherapy for leukemia. His absolute granulocyte count = 500. Which of the following nursing assessments would be the most important to monitor for the sequelae of prolonged leukopenia?
  A. Presence of fever.
  B. Presence of tissue swelling.
  C. Presence of localized pus.
  D. Presence of localized pain.

90. Which of the following chemotherapy agents has a greater risk for causing stomatitis?
  A. 5-fluorouracil.
  B. Dacarbazine.
  C. Cisplatin.
  D. Vinblastine.

91. Which of the following regimens would you recommend to a patient at risk for developing stomatitis?
  A. Schedule oral care q 2 hr with a soft toothbrush and nonfluoridated abrasive dentifrice to remove debris.
  B. Rinse mouth q 2 hr while awake and q 4 hr during the night with a baking soda and peroxide rinse.
  C. Schedule oral care q 2–4 hr while awake with a soft toothbrush, fluoridated toothpaste, and oral irrigations of baking soda, salt, and water.
  D. Continue with current oral care, BID brushing and rinse with commercial rinses until stomatitis actually develops.

92. In teaching Ms. S about her continuous fluorouracil infusion, you have included instructions about the importance of an oral care protocol. These instructions include
  A. perform an assessment of the oral cavity on a weekly basis.
  B. remove white patches gently if present on your tongue or mouth and apply a lanolin-based gel.
  C. begin a low residue, semi-soft diet to prevent stomatitis.
  D. call your doctor immediately if white patches appear on your tongue or mouth.

93. Inflammation of the membranes of the oral cavity is called
  A. esophagitis.
  B. stomatitis.
  C. xerostomia.
  D. herpes simplex.

86.   *Answer:* **A**

Rationale: Bringing pictures of the dog to the hospital is the only action that limits direct exposure of Mr. S to potential carriers of exogenous organisms.

87.   *Answer:* **C**

Rationale: Immunizations are discouraged when the patient is immunocompromised. However, Graze (1980) indicated antibacterial vaccines may be given when the absolute granulocyte count is normal.

88.   *Answer:* **C**

Rationale: Avoid trauma to the oral mucosa; therefore, flossing should be eliminated. Decreasing the frequency of hair washing will not minimize or prevent hair loss. The use of an electric razor is recommended for shaving. Because the majority of infections in immunocompromised patients are from endogenous organisms, handwashing is the most important self-care measure.

89.   *Answer:* **A**

Rationale: In the case of a patient with both immature (leukemia) and inadequate numbers (nadir from chemotherapy) of

granulocytes, the local symptoms of infection— redness, swelling, pain, and pus—may not be present. Therefore, the most important sign would be fever.

90.   *Answer:* **A**

Rationale: 5-fluorouracil is a chemotherapy drug associated with a high incidence of stomatitis. It interferes with the normal replacement of epithelial cells.

91.   *Answer:* **C**

Rationale: This is the least abrasive and most effective program. It is done routinely and contains no abrasive or drying agents that could promote stomatitis.

92.   *Answer:* **D**

Rationale: White patches indicate an infectious process (usually fungal) and can be serious if not treated. Oral assessment should be done at least once daily. White patches should never be removed. Diet will not prevent stomatitis.

93.   *Answer:* **B**

Rationale: This is the definition of stomatitis.

94. Mrs. B is currently receiving radiation therapy to the chest wall for locally recurrent breast cancer. She complains of pain while swallowing, burning, and tightness in her chest. These symptoms may indicate
A. radiation enteritis.
B. esophagitis.
C. hiatal hernia.
D. stomatitis.

95. Mrs. L is experiencing esophagitis secondary to her radiation therapy. Which of the following comments indicate that she needs more instruction about the management of esophagitis?
A. "I guess I'll be eating bland food for awhile."
B. "It's a good thing I like pudding!"
C. "I know to avoid milk since it will cause phlegm."
D. "So much for the steak dinner we are having tonight!"

96. Ms. S, a normally meticulous woman, presents to the clinic looking disheveled. Physical exam reveals a heart rate of 124 and respiration rate of 30. Her skin is moist and cold. She responds inappropriately to questions and appears emotionally labile. These findings indicate Ms. S is suffering from
A. depression.
B. delirium.
C. anxiety.
D. schizophrenia.

97. The family of Ms. S reports that, since the initiation of narcotic analgesics, she has had some noticeable changes in behavior. Which of the following could also be a factor in behavioral changes?
A. Hypercalcemia.
B. Metastasis to the adrenal glands.
C. Aminoglycoside therapy.
D. Long-term oral cyclophosphamide.

98. Which of Ms. S's daughter's statements indicate her understanding of her mother's care?
A. "If Mother's behavior changes, I know to stop her pain medication immediately."
B. "I'm so glad she is on her new pain medicine, and we don't have to worry about her behavior changes anymore."
C. "We've arranged a big surprise homecoming party for Mother."
D. "We're going to keep things quiet at home for awhile. We have asked all but a few close friends to refrain from visiting for now."

99. Ms. J calls you to report that her husband, who has colon cancer, is acting very strangely. He is sleeping more and, when awake, has periods of confusion. At his clinic appointment you notice his sclera are jaundiced and his abdomen is enlarged. The most likely cause of his delirium is
A. sepsis.
B. narcotic toxicity.
C. hepatic failure.
D. hypoxia.

100. Signs and symptoms of progressive delirium do **NOT** include
A. agitation.
B. withdrawal.
C. hallucinations.
D. delusions.

101. Mrs. B is to be discharged after a ten-day hospital course for combination chemotherapy and radiation therapy. A constant complaint has been overwhelming fatigue. Which of the following comments indicate that she is beginning to alter her lifestyle to compensate for her fatigue?
A. "I'll be glad to be home and back in the swing of things. I'll be fine."
B. "My family will be so glad to have me home. They haven't had a decent meal since I've been here."
C. "My church has offered to make us dinner a few nights a week. Maybe I should take them up on their offer now."
D. "I've got to be strong for my kids. They need me the way I used to be. They need a real mom."

102. Which of the following symptoms of Mr. B does **NOT** mandate notification of the health care team?
A. Pallor, tachycardia, and dizziness.
B. Sudden onset of lethargy.
C. Increased need for rest periods during the day.
D. Unresolved depression.

94. *Answer:* **B**

Rationale: Difficulty in swallowing, pain and tightness in the chest are signs of esophagitis.

95. *Answer:* **C**

Rationale: Milk does not "cause" phlegm; dairy products may cause thickened secretions in some patients, but not in all cases. Milk products coat and protect the mucosa.

96. *Answer:* **B**

Rationale: Tachycardia, tachypnea, moist skin, and disorientation are classic symptoms of delirium.

97. *Answer:* **A**

Rationale: Hypercalcemia can cause confusion.

98. *Answer:* **D**

Rationale: A calm, familiar environment is important for patients suffering from delirium because they have an increased sensitivity to their environment.

99. *Answer:* **C**

Rationale: Hepatic toxicity can cause delirium and is characterized by jaundice, ascites, and changes in behavior.

100. *Answer:* **B**

Rationale: Withdrawal is an early sign of delirium.

101. *Answer:* **C**

Rationale: Patients need to begin to ask for assistance and explore energy-saving activities during treatment.

102. *Answer:* **C**

Rationale: Taking rest periods during the day is common for persons experiencing treatment-related fatigue.

103.   Mrs. B tells you she feels inadequate as a wife and mother because she can no longer carry out her usual household functions with the same energy as before she started radiation. What advice would you give Mrs. B?
- A.   "Prioritize your activities. Elicit help from family and friends."
- B.   "Reassign all of your household activities to other family members."
- C.   "Ignore the household chores. They will be there when you get better."
- D.   "Don't worry, everyone gets a little tired from therapy."

104. Mrs. B is currently receiving radiation therapy as treatment for breast cancer. She complains of apathy, impaired concentration, and feeling increasingly tired, yet sleeping longer. These complaints suggest Mrs. B is experiencing
- A.   hyponatremia.
- B.   fatigue.
- C.   hypocalcemia.
- D.   radiation pneumonitis.

105. Mrs. B is receiving radiation therapy. Which of the following conditions would increase her sense of fatigue?
- A.   Anemia.
- B.   Thrombocytopenia.
- C.   Hyperkalemia.
- D.   Hypernatremia.

106. Ms. F complains of inability to carry out her daily activities. She becomes tired very easily. Her Hgb is 7.5. The most relevant nursing diagnosis would be activity intolerance related to
- A.   decreased tissue perfusion.
- B.   dehydration.
- C.   depression.
- D.   leukopenia.

107. Mr. P is a 70-year-old man with colon cancer who needs assistance with his personal care. He has no skilled needs, so Medicare will not cover the cost of care. He wants to remain home and calls you for assistance. Which of the following organizations would be an appropriate referral?
- A.   Leukemia Society of America.
- B.   American Cancer Society.
- C.   Candlelighters.
- D.   I Can Cope.

108. Ms. S, an 82-year-old woman with metastatic breast cancer, has been refusing visiting-nurse services despite increasing difficulties managing her personal care. She has lived alone all of her life, and her family is concerned about her. Your first action would be to
- A.   explore the patient's feelings about dependence and independence.
- B.   suggest nursing home placement to the family.
- C.   threaten the patient with readmission to hospital.
- D.   counsel the family not to interfere with the patient's chosen lifestyle.

109. Among persons with cancer, the highest disease-related risk for constipation is
- A.   neurotoxic effects of tumor enzymes.
- B.   neurogenic effects of paraneoplastic syndromes.
- C.   obstructive effects of tumor growth.
- D.   gastrocolic reflex inhibition by tumor secretions.

110. Which of the following interventions for constipation is most likely to interfere with normal physiological functioning of the bowel and lead to dependency?
- A.   Stool softeners.
- B.   Stool expanders.
- C.   Fiber supplements.
- D.   Laxatives.

111. Implementation of a bowel program is indicated in patients regularly receiving which of the following?
- A.   Chemotherapeutic agents.
- B.   Narcotic analgesics.
- C.   Nutritional supplements.
- D.   Tranquilizers.

112. A bowel-elimination program includes a minimum daily fluid intake of
- A.   1000 ml.
- B.   2000 ml.
- C.   3000 ml.
- D.   4000 ml.

103. *Answer:* **A**

Rationale: Persons experiencing fatigue need to prioritize activities and learn to ask others for help. Because Mrs. B's sense of worth is tied to her role as wife and mother, you would not wish to take *all* these activities away from her.

104. *Answer:* **B**

Rationale: Impaired concentration, apathy, and feelings of tiredness, despite increased hours of sleep, all indicate fatigue, a common complaint of persons on radiation therapy.

105. *Answer:* **A**

Rationale: Fatigue is a symptom of anemia.

106. *Answer:* **A**

Rationale: Lowered Hgb results in decreased tissue perfusion, which leads to decreased activity tolerance.

107. *Answer:* **B**

Rationale: The ACS often has grants or services to assist with care at home.

108. *Answer:* **A**

Rationale: Patients often have difficulties accepting help from others.

109. *Answer:* **C**

Rationale: Responses other than C may be remotely possible, but they do not account for the *highest* disease-related risk.

110. *Answer:* **D**

Rationale: The prevention of dependency on drugs for bowel control is a nursing goal.

111. *Answer:* **B**

Rationale: Prevention of constipation is an important component of the role of the nurse. Constipation is often a side effect of narcotics.

112. *Answer:* **C**

Rationale: Adequate fluid intake is essential in the prevention of constipation and patient discomfort; 3000 ml is commonly accepted as the goal.

113. A rectal digital examination to check for a fecal impaction is contraindicated if the patient is
    A. febrile.
    B. anemic.
    C. dehydrated.
    D. thrombocytopenic.

114. A critical change in the condition of a patient with constipation that should be reported to the physician is
    A. inadequate fluid intake.
    B. absence of bowel sounds.
    C. cramping with enemas.
    D. failure to evacuate daily.

115. Which would be correct nutritional advice for a patient prone to constipation?
    A. Keep foods soft and bland to avoid bowel irritation.
    B. Take all narcotics with milk to reduce the incidence of GI upset.
    C. Maintain fluid intake of 1000 cc/day to prevent dehydration.
    D. Include foods high in fiber and roughage in daily diet.

116. Which medication could cause constipation?
    A. Chloralhydrate.
    B. Digoxin.
    C. Morphine.
    D. Daunorubicin.

117. Ms. C complains of abdominal bloating and cramping with no bowel movement for five days. She usually has a bowel movement every day. Bowel sounds are present. She received 80 mg of adriamycin ten days prior to this appointment. Recommendations include
    A. a soap-suds enema to relieve constipation immediately.
    B. a Fleet enema to stimulate peristalsis.
    C. an oral cathartic until bowel movement, then evaluate the need for daily stool softeners.
    D. beginning daily stool softeners for constipation and mild narcotic for abdominal pain.

118. Which class of chemotherapy drugs can cause constipation?
    A. Antibiotics.
    B. Antimetabolites.
    C. Vinca alkaloids.
    D. Alkylating agents.

119. Mr. F is receiving combination therapy of 5-fluorouracil and radiation for colorectal cancer. He is most at risk for which of the following side effects?
    A. Peripheral neuropathy.
    B. Alopecia.
    C. Thrombocytopenia.
    D. Diarrhea.

120. A nursing diagnosis related to diarrhea is alteration in protective mechanisms related to altered skin integrity. Which of the following nursing actions would correspond to this diagnosis?
    A. Applying zinc oxide ointment to rectal area to protect skin.
    B. Applying a skin-barrier dressing to rectal area to form protective barrier.
    C. Avoiding sitz baths—they will promote bacterial growth.
    D. Cleansing rectal area with water and mild soap after each bowel movement, rinsing well, and patting dry.

121. Diarrhea can lead to fluid and electrolyte imbalance. Which of the following imbalances is of particular concern?
    A. Hypokalemia.
    B. Hypercalcemia.
    C. Hypernatremia.
    D. Hyperkalemia.

122. Mrs. S is receiving radiation therapy to her abdomen and asks for dietary instructions to decrease her diarrhea. You instruct her as follows:
    A. eat a high-fiber diet that is high in protein.
    B. eat what you want because diet has little or no impact on radiation-induced diarrhea.
    C. begin a low-residue diet that is high in protein.
    D. avoid solid foods and begin supplemental liquid feedings until diarrhea resolves.

113. *Answer:* **D**

Rationale: Digital rectal examination may cause abrasion, leading to bleeding in thrombocytopenic patients.

114. *Answer:* **B**

Rationale: Absence of bowel sounds may be a sign of obstruction, which is a potentially life-threatening complication.

115. *Answer:* **D**

Rationale: Fluid intake should be 3000 cc and diet should be high in fiber and roughage to stimulate peristalsis.

116. *Answer:* **C**

Rationale: Narcotics can cause constipation.

117. *Answer:* **C**

Rationale: Constipation of three days or more is unusual in this patient and demands immediate relief. Patients ten-days post adriamycin are susceptible to infection and should avoid rectal medications or treatments.

118. *Answer:* **C**

Rationale: Vinca alkaloids can cause toxicity of the smooth muscle of the GI tract, leading to reduced peristalsis.

119. *Answer:* **D**

Rationale: Combined 5-fluorouracil and abdominal radiation therapy have a synergistic effect to cause diarrhea.

120. *Answer:* **D**

Rationale: The rectal area needs to be cleansed and dried to inhibit growth of bacteria. Sitz baths promote comfort.

121. *Answer:* **A**

Rationale: Diarrhea results in potassium loss.

122. *Answer:* **C**

Rationale: A low-residue diet will decrease irritation of the GI tract.

123. Which of the following classes of chemotherapy drugs carries a high-risk potential for diarrhea?
   A. Vinca alkaloids.
   B. Antimetabolites.
   C. Hormonal agents.
   D. Nitrosureas.

124. Which of the following is **NOT** a potential cause of urinary incontinence?
   A. Fluid overload.
   B. Sedation.
   C. Fecal impaction.
   D. Spinal cord compression.

125. Ms. L is at the nadir of her chemotherapy regimen. She is occasionally incontinent of urine, and her family requests a Foley catheter be inserted. You explain this would not be wise at this time because
   A. Ms. L is at increased risk for infection.
   B. it would be difficult for Ms. L to regain her bladder function.
   C. Ms. L needs to become more independent with her daily activities.
   D. the insertion of a Foley catheter would delay Ms. L's discharge.

126. Mrs. S is an elderly, alert female with metastatic breast cancer. She was admitted to your unit for management of treatment-induced congestive heart failure. Upon admission she is given 80 mg of furosemide. Since she is elderly, frail, and in a strange environment, you are concerned about urinary incontinence. Your nursing plan would include
   A. providing adult diapers for the patient so she will not have to worry about incontinence.
   B. inserting a Foley catheter to avoid incontinence.
   C. placing a commode at the bedside and instructing the patient in its use.
   D. no special measures.

127. Mrs. P is going home after a stay on the rehab unit. She will be performing intermittent self-catheterization. Her discharge instructions include which of the following?
   A. Use a new catheter with each catheterization.
   B. Perform catheterization only when you feel the urge to void.
   C. Expect scant amount of blood in the urine as normal and no cause for alarm.
   D. Use catheters repeatedly as long as they are cleansed after each use.

128. Which of the following nursing diagnoses would be *least applicable* to a patient with an indwelling Foley catheter?
   A. Potential body image disturbance.
   B. Alteration in skin integrity.
   C. Alteration in elimination due to incontinence.
   D. Alteration in fluid balance.

129. Mrs. P has urinary incontinence related to a central neurological deficit. You are to begin a bladder training program with her in anticipation of discharge. Which of the following measures would be included in your program?
   A. Maintain fluid intake at 1000–1500 cc/day.
   B. Avoid measures that would artificially stimulate voiding.
   C. Establish a voiding schedule, offering the bedpan every two hours.
   D. Avoid intermittent catheterization to prevent infection.

130. Mrs. J, a 32-year-old woman, is scheduled to receive external radiation therapy and a cesium implant for cancer of the cervix. Which of the following statements would be most accurate in teaching Mrs. J about the potential effects of radiation therapy on sexuality?
   A. "You will continue to have normal menstrual periods during treatment."
   B. "You may notice some vaginal dryness after treatment is completed."
   C. "You should avoid penile–vaginal intercourse during treatment."
   D. "You may notice some vaginal relaxation after treatment is completed."

123. *Answer:* **B**

Rationale: Gastrointestinal alterations are a common toxicity of antimetabolites.

124. *Answer:* **A**

Rationale: Persons with normal bladder control can handle increased fluids without incontinence.

125. *Answer:* **A**

Rationale: Indwelling Foley catheters are a source of infection.

126. *Answer:* **C**

Rationale: The patient should be near a commode for easy access and for measurement of urine output.

127. *Answer:* **D**

Rationale: Self-intermittent-catheterization is a clean, not sterile, technique.

128. *Answer:* **D**

Rationale: The insertion of a Foley catheter is a measure to maintain fluid balance.

129. *Answer:* **C**

Rationale: A schedule is an integral part of a bladder training program. The program also includes teaching measures to stimulate voiding and catheterizing patient until residual is less than 50 cc after voiding.

130. *Answer:* **B**

Rationale: Radiation fields that include the ovaries usually result in premature menopause. Without estrogen replacement, vaginal dryness will result.

131. As a nurse caring for Mr. C, subsequent to an abdominoperineal resection, which of the following patient/significant-other concerns are most realistic to discuss with him?
   A. Awareness of a variety of ways for sexual pleasure.
   B. Ability to ejaculate with intercourse.
   C. Security in his masculinity after surgery.
   D. Ability to achieve an erection after surgery.

132. Mrs. J is receiving radiation therapy for vaginal cancer. Which of the following actions is most likely to decrease dyspareunia after therapy?
   A. Use of a vaginal dilator with petroleum jelly lubrication three times a week.
   B. Use of a vaginal estrogen cream as lubrication with intercourse.
   C. Male-on-top positioning for penile–vaginal intercourse.
   D. Waiting three months before resuming penile–vaginal intercourse.

133. Mrs. J is scheduled to have a mastectomy for breast cancer. Which of the following questions would be **MOST** appropriate for the nurse to ask when discussing the potential impact of surgery on sexuality?
   A. "Do you have any concerns about how the loss of your breast may affect how others see you?"
   B. "Some women have concerns about the effects the surgery will have on their sexual life. Do you have any concerns?"
   C. "Do you have any problems with your sexual life at this time?"
   D. "Some women don't see themselves as feminine after surgery. Do you?"

134. Mrs. G has been told to use a vaginal dilator following radiation therapy to the cervix. Which of the following statements is most appropriate for the nurse to use in teaching Mrs. G?
   A. Insert the dilator into your vagina as quickly as possible.
   B. Lubricate the dilator with an oil-based jelly.
   C. Leave the dilator inserted for 10 minutes each time.
   D. Wait six weeks after radiation to begin using the dilator.

135. Mrs. T is receiving radiation therapy to the pelvis. She states that she has not had intercourse for several weeks, although she desires sexual intimacy. Which of the following suggestions would be most appropriate for the nurse to make to Mrs. T?
   A. Let your partner know you are interested in having sex.
   B. Limit the amount of time you and your partner initially spend on intercourse.
   C. Ask your partner why he hasn't wanted to have sex.
   D. Concentrate on pleasing your partner during intercourse.

136. Mr. G reports that he is unable to achieve a firm erection. He is two years post radiation to the pelvis. The doctor has discussed the option of a penile implant. Which of the following comments made by Mr. G would indicate a need for additional information?
   A. "When erect, my penis probably won't be as long."
   B. "Most men and their partners are satisfied with the function of the penile implants."
   C. "I may need to wear an athletic supporter to conceal the semi-rigid rod implant."
   D. "I may penetrate immediately since my penis is erect."

131. *Answer:* **A**

Rationale: With an abdominoperineal resection, the patient most likely will not be able to sustain an erection and will have retrograde ejaculation. Internalization of the impact of these changes on the patient's self-concept most likely will not occur prior to leaving the hospital.

132. *Answer:* **B**

Rationale: Radiation therapy will limit the production of estrogen by the ovaries; vaginal dryness and fragility result. The application of vaginal estrogen cream will minimize these symptoms.

133. *Answer:* **B**

Rationale: The correct answer provides permission for sexual concerns. By using "some women. . .," an opportunity is provided for the patient to express her individual concerns.

134. *Answer:* **C**

Rationale: The vaginal dilator is used to maintain the vaginal space and minimize the stenotic effects of radiation therapy. However, the effectiveness of the intervention depends on the correct technique and consistency of use.

135. *Answer:* **A**

Rationale: Often the partner is reluctant to initiate sexual activities for fear of hurting the patient or because they make an assumption that the patient does not want to have sex.

136. *Answer:* **D**

Rationale: Although the penis is erect, the male is advised to engage in foreplay to achieve a level of excitement prior to penetration.

137. Mrs. R had a below-the-knee amputation one month ago for sarcoma. She has refused to look at the surgical site. Such behavior is most suggestive of a disturbance in
  A. self-esteem.
  B. body-image.
  C. role performance.
  D. self-identity.

138. A primary objective of a patient visit by a trained volunteer who has adjusted successfully to a similar experience, such as the Reach to Recovery program for mastectomy patients, is to promote adaptation to changes in
  A. body structure and functioning by discussing prostheses, clothing, and appearance.
  B. prognosis and life expectancy by discussing the similarity of the visitor's and patient's disease.
  C. role functioning and lifestyle by discussing vocational rehabilitation and other services available.
  D. sexual and social functioning by discussing personal changes in sexual or social functioning.

139. Persons with body-image disturbances are frequently found to exhibit self-destructive behavior. In dealing with such behavior, the primary goal of the nurse is to assist the patient to identify
  A. moral implications of the behavior.
  B. psychological basis for the behavior.
  C. logical basis for the behavior.
  D. adverse effects of the behavior.

140. Early postoperative dismissal of individuals undergoing a mastectomy is an example of one change in the health care system which makes it more difficult to plan and implement postoperative teaching. Which characteristic of the learner maximizes teaching outcomes?
  A. Mental capacity to learn.
  B. Motivation to learn.
  C. Readiness to learn.
  D. Desire to learn.

141. The nurse who identifies characteristics of body-image dysfunction in an individual who has a diagnosis or treatment that involves structure or function of the reproductive system should approach the subject by
  A. giving the patient permission to discuss sexual concerns.
  B. providing literature on normal sexual structure and function.
  C. initiating a referral for sexual counseling.
  D. providing intensive sexual counseling.

142. Which of the following patient outcome behaviors represents the highest level of adaptation to body-image changes?
  A. Discusses changes in body structure and function.
  B. Lists emergency resources to deal with self-destructive behavior.
  C. Serves as a volunteer in a patient-to-patient visitation program.
  D. Discusses plans to return to previous work role.

143. Mrs. J is being treated with fluoxymesterone (Halotestin) for breast cancer. Which of the following changes might be expected as a side effect?

  A. Decreased libido.
  B. Deepening of voice.
  C. Breast tenderness.
  D. Hair loss.

144. Mrs. K is a 24-year-old woman who was recently diagnosed with Hodgkin's disease. She and her husband had been trying to start a family. Which of the following statements, if made by Mr. K, would indicate a need for further sexual counseling?
  A. "We will have to postpone starting our family."
  B. "She won't be able to get pregnant while on chemotherapy."
  C. "Even though she is on chemotherapy, we will be able to have intercourse."
  D. "We need to talk about how we feel about the changes in her appearance."

137. *Answer:* **B**

Rationale: Body image is more focused than concepts of self or role.

138. *Answer:* **A**

Rationale: Response A delineates the limits of the volunteer's role. Prognosis, personal diseases, or sexual counseling are beyond the scope of responsibility for volunteers.

139. *Answer:* **D**

Rationale: The adverse effects of body-image disturbances have implications for patient safety and should be given priority. Attention to adverse effects is a response that can be an independent nursing role. Other responses refer to interventions that are not necessarily appropriate or are representative of the role of other health professionals.

140. *Answer:* **C**

Rationale: The timing of patient teaching is influenced more by the health care system than by principles of learning. Nurses must adapt to the system, yet be resourceful in facilitating learning. Readiness to learn is an important concept to apply.

141. *Answer:* **A**

Rationale: This response encourages the respondent to apply the PLISSIT (permission, limited information, specific suggestions, and intensive therapy) model of sexual counseling to patients who have body-image disturbances related to sexual functioning. The first step is "permission giving," which is reflected in the first response.

142. *Answer:* **C**

Rationale: The third response represents actual, rather than planned, reintegration with constructive channeling of energies; therefore, C represents a higher level of adaptation than attention to safety (B), knowledge (A), or planned activity (D).

143. *Answer:* **B**

Rationale: Fluoxymesterone (Halotestin) is an androgen, and long-term usage will result in masculinizing effects, including deepening of the voice, hirsutism, and increased libido.

144. *Answer:* **B**

Rationale: Although chemotherapy will decrease the maturation of ova, pregnancy may occur and birth control should be used since teratogenic effects are associated with antineoplastic agents.

145. Mr. J is scheduled to begin chemotherapy for Hodgkin's disease. He is concerned about the effects of chemotherapy on sexual functioning. Which of the following statements, if made by Mr. J, would indicate a need for additional counseling?
  A. "Chemotherapy can result in a marked decrease in the number of sperm."
  B. "I may notice a change in my desire for sex while I am on chemotherapy."
  C. "Chemotherapy will cause me to feel more tired and perhaps lose interest in sex."
  D. "I will not need to use a condom for birth control after I begin chemotherapy."

146. Mr. G is anticipating storing his sperm. Which of the following statements, if made by Mr. G, would indicate a need for further teaching?
  A. "I will need to collect the sperm for storing prior to beginning treatment."
  B. "I will need to collect my sperm only once."
  C. "I will have a test to determine the number of sperm I have before collecting."
  D. "I will have to masturbate to collect the sperm."

147. The types of chemotherapeutic agents most often recognized as having long-term reproductive effects are
  A. nitrosoureas.
  B. alkylating agents.
  C. antitumor antibiotics.
  D. all of the above.

148. Which of the following positions would be most beneficial in decreasing the work of breathing?
  A. Sitting in a chair with shoulders erect and pushed backward.
  B. Sitting in a chair with shoulders relaxed and rolled forward.
  C. Sitting in bed with the head of the bed elevated twenty-five degrees.
  D. Sitting in bed with the head of the bed elevated seventy-five degrees.

149. Which of the following breathing techniques is most likely to improve the efficiency of Mr. S's breathing?
  A. Exhaling through the nose.
  B. Exhaling through pursed lips.
  C. Exhaling one-half as long as inhaling.
  D. Exhaling using accessory muscles.

150. Which of the following assessments would be most accurate in evaluating the severity of Mrs. J's dyspnea?
  A. Respiratory rate and depth.
  B. Use of accessory muscles for breathing.
  C. Ability of Mrs. J to accomplish activities of daily living.
  D. Mrs. J's perception of the amount of difficulty in breathing.

151. In preparing Mrs. C, a patient experiencing dyspnea, for discharge from the hospital, the nurse evaluates the effectiveness of patient/family teaching. Which of the following statements, if made by Mrs. C, would indicate a need for additional teaching?
  A. "If I have trouble breathing, I will just lie down with my head elevated on several pillows."
  B. "I will keep the temperature in the house a few degrees higher than usual."
  C. "I will arrange for a friend to be available if I need someone."
  D. "If I notice a big change in my dyspnea, I will call my doctor."

152. Which of the following dietary recommendations should the nurse make to increase the intake of nutrients needed for erythropoiesis?
  A. Milk, eggs, liver, and green leafy vegetables.
  B. Apples, peanuts, oats, and cottage cheese.
  C. Cantaloupe, lima beans, and sweet potatoes.
  D. Dry yeast, grapefruit, and tuna fish.

145. *Answer:* **D**

Rationale: Although the number of sperm will be markedly decreased, birth control should not be discontinued during therapy due to the potential teratogenic effects of chemotherapy.

146. *Answer:* **B**

Rationale: Samples with an adequate number of sperm, to allow for loss during the freezing and thawing process, require several collections, 24–48 hours apart.

147. *Answer:* **B**

Rationale: Alkylating agents can cause permanent injury to the gonads. Primary ovarian failure, with amenorrhea, decreased estradiol, and elevated gonadotropins, has been reported in women of all ages. In men, damage to the germinal epithelium of the testes, with decreased or absent spermatogenesis, can occur.

148. *Answer:* **B**

Rationale: The work of breathing is reduced by decreasing the resistance against which the respiratory muscles must work.

149. *Answer:* **B**

Rationale: Dyspnea is a distressing and powerless experience for patients. Concrete nursing interventions to modify the experience of, and the reaction to, dyspnea are important. With pursed-lip breathing, back pressure is created to keep airways open. This promotes more complete exhalation and facilitates removal of secretions from the tracheobronchial tree.

150. *Answer:* **D**

Rationale: Dyspnea is a subjective complaint. Other parameters may be indices of the compromise of oxygenation and endurance, but patient perception of severity is the most accurate.

151. *Answer:* **B**

Rationale: Breathing is easier in a cooler environment.

152. *Answer:* **A**

Rationale: Foods high in protein, vitamin B_{12}, folic acid, and iron are needed for erythropoiesis.

153. Mrs. M has completed a six-week course of radiation therapy to the mediastinum. She currently has a hemoglobin of 7.5. In evaluating the effectiveness of discharge teaching, which of the following comments, if made by Mrs. M, would indicate a need for additional instruction?
   A. "I should eat foods high in protein, iron, and vitamin B_{12}."
   B. "If I notice any dizziness, I should avoid driving the car."
   C. "I may not be able to do all my housework and go to work too."
   D. "If I notice any palpitations, I will just lie down for awhile."

154. Mrs. J has a hemoglobin of 6.5. She is experiencing symptoms of cerebral tissue hypoxia. Which of the following nursing interventions would be most important in providing care for Mrs. J?
   A. Providing rest periods throughout the day.
   B. Instituting energy conservation techniques.
   C. Assisting in ambulation to bathroom.
   D. Checking temperature of water prior to bathing.

155. Mrs. C is receiving radiation therapy to the pelvis for cancer of the cervix. Her hemoglobin is 7.0. Which of the following complaints expressed by Mrs. C would be indicative of tissue hypoxia related to anemia?
   A. Dizziness.
   B. Fatigue relieved by rest.
   C. Skin that is warm to the touch.
   D. Apathy.

153. *Answer:* **D**

Rationale: Palpitation is a significant change in the condition of the patient and may be indicative of progressing anemia. Therefore, the patient should report the symptom to the physician.

154. *Answer:* **C**

Rationale: Cerebral tissue hypoxia is commonly associated with dizziness. The greatest risk to the client with dizziness is potential injury, especially with changes in position.

155. *Answer:* **A**

Rationale: Cerebral tissue hypoxia is commonly associated with dizziness. Recognition of cerebral hypoxia is critical since the body will attempt to shunt oxygenated blood to vital organs.

REFERENCES

Alexander EJ, (1991). Injury, Potential For, Related to Thrombocytopenia, in, McNally JC, Somerville ET, Miaskowski C, Rostad M, (eds). *Guidelines for Cancer Nursing Practice,* (2nd ed). Philadelphia: WB Saunders, pp. 203–207.

Benner P, (1991). Stress and Coping with Cancer, in, Baird SB, McCorkle R, Grant M, (eds). Cancer Nursing A Comprehensive Textbook. Philadelphia: W. B. Saunders Company, pp. 74–81.

Brager BL, Yasko JM, (1984). Care of the Client Receiving Chemotherapy. Reston, VA: Reston Publishing Co., Inc.

Brown M, Kiss M, Outlaw E, Viamontes C, (1986). *Standards of Oncology Nursing Practice.* New York, NY: John Wiley and Sons.

Campbell BK, (1984). Anxiety, in, Jacobs MM, Geels W.(eds). *Signs and Symptoms in Nursing: Interpretation and Management.* Philadelphia: JB Lippincott.

Carnevali DL, Reiner AC, (1990). *The Cancer Experience: Nursing Diagnosis and Management.* Philadelphia: JB Lippincott.

Carpenito LJ, (1983). *Nursing Diagnosis: Application to Clinical Practice.* Philadelphia: JB Lippincott.

Carpenito LJ, (1989). *Handbook of Nursing Diagnosis.* Philadelphia: JB Lippincott.

Carrieri VK, Janson-Bjerklie S, (1986). Dyspnea, in, Carrieri VK, Lindsey AM, West CM, (eds). *Pathophysiological Phenomena in Nursing.* Philadelphia: WB Saunders, pp. 191–218.

Childs CC, Traverna M, (1990). Hospice Care, in, Groenwald SL, Frogge MH, Goodman M, Yarbro CH, (eds). *Cancer Nursing Principles and Practice,* (2nd ed). Boston: Jones and Bartlett, pp. 1132–1149.

Clark JC, (1990). Psychosocial Dimensions: The Patient, in Groenwald SL, Frogge MH, Goodman M, Yarbro CH, (eds). *Cancer Nursing Principles and Practice,* (2nd ed). Boston: Jones and Bartlett, pp. 346–364.

Clark JC, McGee RF, (1992). Nursing Management of Responses to the Cancer Experience, in, Clark JC, McGee RF, (eds). *Core Curriculum for Oncology Nursing,* (2nd ed). Philadelphia: W B Saunders.

Coyle N, Foley KM, (1991). Alterations in Comfort: Pain, in, Baird SB, McCorkle R, Grant M, (eds). *Cancer Nursing A Comprehensive Textbook.* Philadelphia: W. B. Saunders Company, pp. 782–805.

Daeffler RJ, Petrosino BM, (1990). *Manual of Oncology Nursing Practice.* Rockville, MD: Aspen Publishers.

Dietz KA, Flaherty AM, (1990). Oncologic Emergencies, in, Groenwald SL, Frogge MH, Goodman M, Yarbro CH, (eds). *Cancer Nursing Principles and Practice,* (2nd ed). Boston: Jones and Bartlett, pp. 644–668.

Dudas S, (1990). Altered Body Image and Sexuality, in Groenwald SL, Frogge MH, Goodman M, Yarbro CH, (eds). *Cancer Nursing Principles and Practice,* (2nd ed). Boston: Jones and Bartlett, pp. 581–593.

Ferrell B, Wisdom C, Wenzl C, Brown J, (1989). Effects of Controlled-release Morphine on Quality of Life for Cancer Pain. *Oncology Nursing Forum,* 16 (4): 521–526.

Goodman M, Harte N, (1990). Breast Cancer, in, Groenwald SL, Frogge MH, Goodman M, Yarbro CH, (eds). *Cancer Nursing Principles and Practice,* (2nd ed). Boston: Jones and Bartlett, pp. 722–750.

Grant M, Ropka ME, (1991). Alterations in Nutrition, in Baird SB, McCorkle R, Grant M, (eds). *Cancer Nursing A Comprehensive Textbook.* Philadelphia: W. B. Saunders Company, pp. 717–741.

Graze P, (1980). Bone Marrow Failure: Management of Anemia, Infections, and Bleeding in the Cancer Patient, in, Haskell C, (ed). *Cancer Treatment.* Philadelphia: WB Saunders, pp. 961–983.

Gwin R, (1990). *Sperm Banking: An Option for Men with Cancer.* Atlanta, GA: Emory University Hospital.

Haluber D, Spross JA. (1991). Alterations in Protective Mechanisms: Hematopoiesis and Bone Marrow Depression, in Baird SB, McCorkle R, Grant M, (eds). *Cancer Nursing A Comprehensive Textbook.* Philadelphia: W. B. Saunders Company, pp. 759–781.

Holland JC, Massie MJ, (1899). *Psychiatric Management of Anxiety in Patients with Cancer.* Chicago, IL: Upjohn Co.

Jalowiec A, Dudas S. (1991). Alterations in Patient Coping, in Baird SB, McCorkle R, Grant M, (eds). *Cancer Nursing A Comprehensive Textbook.* Philadelphia: W. B. Saunders Company, p. 806–820.

Johnson BL, Gross J, (eds), (1985). *Handbook of Oncology Nursing.* Bethany, CT: Fleschner Publishing Co.

Kaye P, (1989). *Notes on Symptom Control in Hospice and Palliative Care.* Essex, CT: Hospice Education Institute.

Krebs LU, (1990). Sexual and Reproductive Dysfunction, in, Groenwald SL, Frogge MH, Goodman M, Yarbro CH, (eds). *Cancer Nursing Principles and Practice,* (2nd ed). Boston: Jones and Bartlett, pp. 563–580.

Lamb MA, (1991). Alterations in Sexuality and Sexual Functioning, in, Baird SB, McCorkle R, Grant M, (eds). *Cancer Nursing A Comprehensive Textbook.* Philadelphia: W. B. Saunders Company, pp. 831–849.

Lang-Kummer JM, (1990). Hypercalcemia, in, Groenwald SL, Frogge MH, Goodman M, Yarbro CH, (eds). *Cancer Nursing Principles and Practice,* (2nd ed). Boston: Jones and Bartlett, pp. 520–534.

Legha SS, Hortobagy GN, Benjamin RS, (1987). Anthracyclines, in, Lokich JJ, (ed). *Cancer Chemotherapy by Infusion.* Chicago: Precept Press Inc., pp. 130–144.

Loescher LJ, Welch-McCaffrey D, Leigh SA, et al., (1989). Surviving Adult Cancers (Part I): Physiologic Effects. *Annals of Internal Medicine*. 111: 411–432.

Lucarelli C, (1985). Intractable Hiccups: A Review of Causes and Current Treatment. *Hospital Pharmacy*. 20: 820–822.

Lydon J, Purl S, Goodman M, (1990). Integumentary and Mucous Membrane Alterations, in, Groenwald SL, Frogge MH, Goodman M, Yarbro CH, (eds). *Cancer Nursing Principles and Practice*, (2nd ed). Boston: Jones and Bartlett, pp. 594–643.

Mood, DW, (1991). The Diagnosis of Cancer: A Life Transition, in Baird SB, McCorkle R, Grant M, (eds). *Cancer Nursing A Comprehensive Textbook*. Philadelphia: W. B. Saunders Company, pp. 219–234.

Petrosino BM, Landrum B, Hackbarth A, (1990). Altered Bowel Elimination, in, Deffler RJ, Petrosino BM, (eds). *Manual of Oncology Nursing Practice: Nursing Diagnosis and Care*. Rockville, MD: Aspen Publications, pp. 157–164.

McNally JC, Somerville ET, Miaskowski C, Rostad M, (eds), (1991). Circulation, in, *Guidelines for Oncology Nursing Practice*, (2nd ed). Philadelphia: WB Saunders, pp. 385–426.

McNally JC, Somerville ET, Miaskowski C, Rostad M, (eds), (1991). Coping, in, *Guidelines for Oncology Nursing Practice*, (2nd ed). Philadelphia: WB Saunders, pp. 101–122.

McNally JC, Somerville ET, Miaskowski C, Rostad M, (eds), (1991). Elimination, in, *Guidelines for Oncology Nursing Practice*, (2nd ed). Philadelphia: WB Saunders, pp. 295–336.

McNally JC, Somerville ET, Miaskowski C, Rostad M, (eds), (1991). Nutrition, in, *Guidelines for Oncology Nursing Practice*, (2nd ed). Philadelphia: WB Saunders, pp. 163–188.

McNally JC, Somerville ET, Miaskowski C, Rostad M, (eds), (1991). Ventilation, in, *Guidelines for Oncology*

Nursing Practice, (2nd ed). Philadelphia: WB Saunders, pp. 351–383.

Moore IM, Ruccione K, (1990). Late Effects of Cancer Treatment, in, Groenwald SL, Frogge MH, Goodman M, Yarbro CH, (eds). *Cancer Nursing Principles and Practice,* (2nd ed). Boston: Jones and Bartlett, pp. 669–685.

National Institute of Mental Health. (1991) *Depression: What You Need to Know*. Rockville, MD: D/ART/Public Inquires, NIMH.

Niemeyer M, (1985). Dyspnea, in, Jacobs MM, Geels W, (eds). *Signs and Symptoms in Nursing*. Philadelphia: JB Lippincott, pp. 431–434.

Preston F, Wilfinger C, (1988). *Memory Bank for Chemotherapy*. Baltimore: Williams and Wilkins.

Roberts SL, (1986). *Behavioral Concepts and the Critically Ill Patient*, (2nd ed). Norwalk, CT: Appleton-Century-Crofts.

Schover LR, (1988). *Sexuality and Cancer: For the Woman Who Has Cancer and Her Partner*. Atlanta, GA: American Cancer Society.

Schreiber JA, (1991). Impaired Gas Exchange, in, McNally JC, Somerville ET, Miaskowski C, Rostad M, (eds), *Guidelines for Cancer Nursing Practice*, (2nd ed). Philadelphia: WB Saunders, pp. 364-369.

Spross JA, (1985). Bone Marrow, in, Johnson L, Gross J, (eds). *Handbook of Oncology Nursing*. New York: John Wiley and Sons, pp. 229–252.

Van Hoff D, Rozenweig M, Piccart M, (1982). The Cardiotoxicity of Anticancer Agents. *Seminars in Oncology*. 9 (1): 23.

Walsh J, Persons C, Wick L, (1987). *Manual of Home Health Care Nursing*. Philadelphia: JB Lippincott.

Werner-Beland J, (1980). *Grief Responses to Long-Term Illness and Disability*. Reston, VA: Reston Publishing Co.

Xytex Corporation, (1989). *Sperm Banking*. Atlanta, GA: Author.

Yasko J, (1983). *Guidelines for Cancer Care: Symptom Management*. Reston, VA: Reston Publishing Co.

5
Oncologic Emergencies

Jane C. Hunter and Marilyn A. Kline

Choose the BEST answer for each of the following questions:

1. All of the following represent signs and symptoms of cardiac tamponade **EXCEPT**
   A. retrosternal chest pain.
   B. muffled heart sounds.
   C. increased jugular vein distention.
   D. widening pulse pressure.

2. All of the following pharmaceutical interventions have been used for pericardial sclerosis **EXCEPT**
   A. tetracycline.
   B. thiotepa.
   C. vincristine.
   D. nitrogen mustard.

3. An individual with which cancer is at risk for developing cardiac tamponade?
   A. Lung cancer.
   B. Sarcoma.
   C. Hodgkin's disease.
   D. Colon cancer.

4. What is the most accurate diagnostic test for cardiac tamponade?
   A. CT scan.
   B. Chest x-ray.
   C. Echocardiogram.
   D. EKG.

5. All of the following signs and symptoms are seen in cardiac tamponade **EXCEPT**
   A. dyspnea.
   B. cough.
   C. narrowing pulse pressure.
   D. bradycardia.

6. Disseminated intravascular coagulopathy (DIC) is a clotting disorder frequently seen in patients who have which malignancy?
   A. Multiple myeloma.
   B. Breast cancer.
   C. Leukemia.
   D. Hodgkin's disease.

7. Which condition, other than cancer, may precipitate the onset of DIC?
   A. Immobility.
   B. Antibiotic therapy.
   C. Renal failure.
   D. Gram-negative sepsis.

8. A 70-year-old male with metastatic cancer of the prostate is admitted to the hospital with shaking chills, hematuria, and lower abdominal pain. BP is 90/60, P = 130, and R = 24. Initial laboratory results are: WBC = 10.7, Hct = 24.6, and platelets = 65,000. A nurse making an initial assessment of this patient should suspect which of the following conditions?
   A. Pyelonephritis.
   B. Disseminated intravascular coagulopathy.
   C. Hemorrhagic cystitis.
   D. Obstructive renal calculi.

1. *Answer:* **D**

   Rationale: In cardiac tamponade, there is a narrowing of the pulse pressure (decreased systolic and increased diastolic blood pressure).

2. *Answer:* **C**

   Rationale: Tetracycline, nitrogen mustard, and Thiotepa have been used as sclerosing agents in the treatment of cardiac tamponade.

3. *Answer:* **A**

   Rationale: Lung cancer, breast cancer, leukemia, melanoma, and non-Hodgkin's lymphoma are among the common cancers that can metastasize to the heart.

4. *Answer:* **C**

   Rationale: Echocardiogram is an accurate, noninvasive method to determine pericardial effusion. It can be done quickly and can even be done at the bedside.

5. *Answer:* **D**

   Rationale: Bradycardia is not associated with cardiac tamponade.

6. *Answer:* **C**

   Rationale: DIC is most frequently associated with promyelocytic leukemia, but may occur with any acute leukemia.

7. *Answer:* **D**

   Rationale: Gram-negative sepsis is recognized as a common cause of DIC.

8. *Answer:* **B**

   Rationale: Response C could account for hematuria; responses A and D could account for chills, temperature, and pain. Only response B could account for all the presenting signs and symptoms.

9. A nurse caring for a patient with suspected disseminated intravascular coagulopathy would expect to find which of the following lab results?
   A. Decreased platelets, decreased fibrinogen.
   B. Decreased platelets, increased fibrinogen.
   C. Increased platelets, decreased fibrinogen.
   D. Increased platelets, increased fibrinogen.

10. The **PRIMARY** goal of nursing care of the patient with DIC is to
   A. maintain normal nutritional status.
   B. maintain IV fluids.
   C. prevent further bleeding and trauma.
   D. protect the patient from infection.

11. DIC represents an imbalance of normal coagulation. Which of the following statements best summarizes the characteristics of this condition?
   A. Excessive amounts of clotting factors.
   B. Accelerated coagulation and the formation of excessive thrombin.
   C. Failure of the fibrinolytic system.
   D. Blocked internal pathway of clotting.

12. The most common cause of hypercalcemia among hospitalized patients is
   A. thiazide diuretic therapy.
   B. decreased prostaglandin production.
   C. malignancies with bone metastases.
   D. Paget's disease of the bone.

13. Hypercalcemia is a complication most often seen in which malignancy?
   A. Breast cancer.
   B. Leukemia.
   C. Glioblastoma.
   D. Chondrosarcoma.

14. Nursing care of the patient with bone metastases and hypercalcemia should include increased mobilization and adequate hydration in order to avoid which of the following sequelae?
   A. Skin breakdown with formation of decubiti.
   B. Increased release of calcium from bone.
   C. Susceptibility to infection such as pneumonia.
   D. Loss of function with formation of contractures.

15. Which of the following would most likely result in hypercalcemia?
   A. Decreased prostaglandin secretion.
   B. Rapid increase in serum calcium levels.
   C. Decreased vitamin D metabolites.
   D. Rapid rise of BUN and creatinine.

16. Nursing care for the patient with hypercalcemia should include which of the following measures?
   A. Providing a high-protein, low-salt diet.
   B. Limiting mobility, providing a high-calorie diet.
   C. Increasing hydration, increasing mobility.
   D. Limiting fluid intake, monitoring output.

17. Signs and symptoms related to the syndrome of inappropriate antidiuretic hormone (SIADH) include all of the following **EXCEPT**
   A. serum hyponatremia.
   B. constipation.
   C. fluid retention.
   D. headache.

18. SIADH is associated with all of the following diseases or treatments **EXCEPT**
   A. uterine cancer.
   B. vincristine.
   C. oat cell lung cancer.
   D. cyclophosphamide.

9. *Answer:* **A**

Rationale: Platelet count is decreased due to platelet consumption. Plasma fibrinogen is decreased due to consumption of fibrinogen by the clotting cascade and by fibrinolysis.

10. *Answer:* **C**

Rationale: While the other three goals are important in the care of the patient with DIC, the prevention of further bleeding and trauma is the obvious *primary* goal.

11. *Answer:* **B**

Rationale: The pathophysiology of DIC involves extensive triggering of the coagulation system, which results in abnormal activation of thrombin formation.

12. *Answer:* **C**

Rationale: Hypercalcemia of malignancy is frequently associated with high tumor burden and end stage disease. Patients with lung and breast cancers account for the highest incidence rates. The common metastatic site of breast and lung cancers is bone.

13. *Answer:* **A**

Rationale: Twenty to forty percent of reported cases of hypercalcemia occur in patients with breast cancer.

14. *Answer:* **B**

Rationale: Hypercalcemia is the result of excessive bone resorption and impaired renal calcium excretion. Mobility and weight bearing are advocated.

15. *Answer:* **B**

Rationale: A rapid increase in serum calcium is indicative of hypercalcemia.

16. *Answer:* **C**

Rationale: Both of these interventions will aid in decreasing serum calcium.

17. *Answer:* **B**

Rationale: Primary symptoms of SIADH are manifestations of water intoxication. Symptoms listed in responses A, C, and D are attributed to the effects of cerebral edema.

18. *Answer:* **A**

Rationale: Responses B, C, and D are diseases or treatments associated with SIADH. The symptoms of SIADH must be recognized to ensure early detection and appropriate management.

19. The following are all appropriate interventions for patients with SIADH **EXCEPT**
    A. forcing fluids.
    B. teaching patients signs and symptoms of hyponatremia.
    C. administering intravenous saline solution.
    D. restricting water.

20. A patient diagnosed with lung cancer presents with a weight gain of twenty pounds in two weeks with no edema present. Additional signs and symptoms include mental confusion, lethargy, anorexia, and muscle cramps. Laboratory findings are serum Na = 120, serum osmolality = 250, 24 hr urine sodium = 300, creatinine = 1, and BUN = 20. Based on this information, which oncologic emergency does this patient *most likely* have?
    A. Syndrome of inappropriate antidiuretic hormone.
    B. Septic shock.
    C. Renal failure.
    D. Tumor lysis syndrome.

21. Mrs. L has recently been diagnosed with limited stage small cell lung cancer. Upon admission, hematologic and biochemical parameters are within normal limits. After vigorous intravenous hydration, Mrs. L is found to be lethargic, disoriented, and confused. Mrs. L is most likely exhibiting symptoms of
    A. hypercalcemia.
    B. syndrome of inappropriate antidiuretic hormone.
    C. hypertrophic pulmonary osteoarthropathy.
    D. Horner's syndrome.

22. Management of the patient with SIADH would include all of the following **EXCEPT**
    A. treatment of underlying disease.
    B. daily weights.
    C. forcing fluids.
    D. fluid restriction.

23. Which cancer is associated with a high mortality rate related to septic shock?
    A. Hematologic malignancy.
    B. Lung cancer.
    C. Breast cancer.
    D. Gastrointestinal cancer.

24. A 26-year-old disoriented and irritable man, with Hodgkin's disease and diabetes, is admitted to the hospital. His temperature is 100°F, pulse = 110, BP = 120/40, R = 30, WBC = 500, platelets = 150,000, and urine output is normal and positive for sugar (blood sugar is 190). Which condition would you *most likely* suspect in this patient?
    A. Hypocalcemia.
    B. Disseminated intravascular coagulopathy.
    C. Septic shock (warm stage).
    D. Diabetic shock.

25. Which absolute granulocyte count places a cancer patient at the greatest risk for developing septic shock?
    A. Greater than 1000.
    B. Less than 500.
    C. Greater than 500.
    D. Less than 2500.

26. Sepsis is the underlying cause of which oncologic emergency?
    A. Cardiac tamponade.
    B. Syndrome of inappropriate antidiuretic hormone.
    C. Disseminated intravascular coagulopathy.
    D. Tumor lysis syndrome.

27. Signs and symptoms of late (cold) stage septic shock include all of the following **EXCEPT**
    A. bradycardia.
    B. cold, clammy skin.
    C. mental confusion.
    D. metabolic acidosis.

28. Which cancer does **NOT** place an individual at high risk for developing spinal cord compression?
    A. Brain.
    B. Lung.
    C. Breast.
    D. Prostate.

29. All of the following interventions may be used in the treatment of spinal cord compression **EXCEPT**
    A. steroids.
    B. radiation therapy.
    C. biological response modifiers (BRMs).
    D. laminectomy.

19.   *Answer:* **A**

Rationale: SIADH is essentially manifested by signs of water intoxication. Therefore, response A would be inappropriate management.

20.   *Answer:* **A**

Rationale: These signs and symptoms are most consistent with SIADH.

21.   *Answer:* **B**

Rationale: Paraneoplastic syndrome is often associated with lung cancer, and ectopic hormone syndrome is most often associated with small cell lung cancer. Symptoms of the syndrome may not be apparent until the patient is given excessive fluids. The most common symptoms include hyponatremia, high urine osmolality, lethargy, altered mental status, and, occasionally, coma and seizures.

22.   *Answer:* **C**

Rationale: Responses A, B, and C are examples of appropriate interventions to manage the syndrome of inappropriate antidiuretic hormone.

23.   *Answer:* **A**

Rationale: Persons with hematologic malignancies present with a disease-related immune deficiency that may be further impaired by treatment. This population has an increased susceptibility to septic shock.

24.   *Answer:* **C**

Rationale: The signs and symptoms are those manifested in early septic shock.

25.   *Answer:* **B**

Rationale: An absolute granulocyte count of less than 500 places patients at a higher risk for infection, which may progress to septic shock.

26.   *Answer:* **C**

Rationale: Disseminated intravascular coagulopathy is a complication commonly associated with septic shock.

27.   *Answer:* **A**

Rationale: Responses B, C, and D are signs and symptoms of late shock. Patients who present in this stage require prompt, accurate nursing and medical assessment and intervention. Tachycardia is a symptom of septic shock.

28.   *Answer:* **A**

Rationale: Cancers of breast, lung, and prostate have a natural history of metastases to the spine.

29.   *Answer:* **C**

Rationale: 1. Radiation therapy (B) may be used alone or before surgery. 2. Steroids (A) can reduce spinal cord edema and pain. 3. BRMs (C) are not indicated in spinal cord compression. 4. Decompression by laminectomy (D) or resection of a vertebral body is used as treatment for spinal cord compression if tumor is not responsive to radiation therapy or if disease recurs in an area already treated with radiation therapy.

30. The most common early symptom of spinal cord compression is
    A. motor weakness.
    B. sensory loss.
    C. sexual impotence.
    D. back pain.

31. All of the following interventions are indicated in monitoring for progression of spinal cord compression **EXCEPT**
    A. palpation of bladder for distention.
    B. assessment for increased severity of pain.
    C. observation for peripheral edema.
    D. assessment for decreased coordination.

32. All of the following interventions are important in the planning for home care of patients who have spinal cord compression **EXCEPT**
    A. helping the patient and family focus on realistic goals to maintain independence.
    B. collaborating with physical therapy for evaluation for assistive devices.
    C. consulting a social worker to determine community resources and support groups.
    D. teaching the patient and family to avoid blood pressure and venipuncture in upper extremities.

33. The malignancy associated with superior vena cava syndrome most frequently is
    A. germ cell tumor.
    B. lymphoma.
    C. breast cancer.
    D. lung cancer.

34. Interventions for the management of superior vena cava syndrome (SVCS) include all of the following **EXCEPT**
    A. reassuring that physical appearance will return to normal as SVCS resolves.
    B. monitoring blood pressure every one hour in unaffected arm.

C. administering O_2 by nasal cannula at 2 L/min.
D. elevating head of bed to 60°.

35. Individuals with which of the following cancers are at high risk for developing superior vena cava syndrome?
    A. Lymphoma/lung.
    B. Liver/lymphoma.
    C. Breast/cervical.
    D. GU/GI.

36. What is the single most important sequela that indicates the increasing acuity of SVCS?
    A. Progressive dyspnea.
    B. Visual disturbances.
    C. Irritability.
    D. Headaches.

37. Which of the following is **NOT** an early sign of superior vena cava syndrome?
    A. Nonproductive cough.
    B. Dyspnea.
    C. Blurred vision.
    D. Hoarseness.

38. Tumor lysis syndrome occurs most commonly in persons with which cancer?
    A. Renal cell carcinoma.
    B. Breast cancer.
    C. Pancreatic cancer.
    D. High grade lymphoma.

39. Patients experiencing tumor lysis syndrome may present with which abnormal parameter?
    A. Hypokalemia.
    B. Hypernatremia.
    C. Hypercalcemia.
    D. Hyperkalemia.

30.   *Answer:* **D**

   Rationale: When tumors press on the spinal cord, pain is usually the initial complaint. The other options are late symptoms.

31.   *Answer:* **C**

   Rationale: Peripheral edema is not a progressive motor neurological deficit that can be caused by compression of the spinal cord.

32.   *Answer:* **D**

   Rationale: Helping patients maintain independence with appropriate use of resources is an important goal of nursing care.

33.   *Answer:* **D**

   Rationale: Seventy percent of patients with superior vena cava syndrome have cancer of the lung.

34.   *Answer:* **B**

   Rationale: Procedures that cause constriction in the upper extremities should be avoided because venous return is already compromised in SVCS. Instead, blood pressure should be monitored on the thigh.

35.   *Answer:* **A**

   Rationale: Lung cancer and lymphomas are the most frequent causes of SVCS.

36.   *Answer:* **A**

   Rationale: Progressive dyspnea, indicating airway obstruction, can result in respiratory arrest and death.

37.   *Answer:* **C**

   Rationale: Blurred vision is a sequela of intracranial hypertension. Intracranial hypertension is not a presenting symptom of SVCS.

38.   *Answer:* **D**

   Rationale: Persons who have a high tumor burden are at risk for the development of tumor lysis syndrome because of the large number of cells lysed during therapy.

39.   *Answer:* **D**

   Rationale: When cells are lysed, potassium is released into the bloodstream, causing abnormally high levels of potassium.

Oncologic Emergencies—Questions 69

40. A 38-year-old male with diffuse histiocytic lymphoma is admitted to the hospital on day two of the first cycle of ProMACE-CytaBOM chemotherapy. The patient complains of weakness, muscle cramps, nausea and vomiting, diarrhea, and oliguria. Lab findings are creatinine = 2.2, BUN = 66, calcium = 6.0, phosphorous = 8, potassium = 5.5, and uric acid = 11. EKG changes are evident since last admission. Based on these findings, this patient is *most likely* experiencing which oncologic emergency?
   A. Disseminated intravascular coagulopathy.
   B. Syndrome of inappropriate antidiuretic hormone.
   C. Tumor lysis syndrome.
   D. Cardiac tamponade.

41. An 18-year-old female patient with newly diagnosed acute lymphocytic leukemia, s/p splenectomy, is to receive initial induction chemotherapy. Assessment included the following findings: WBC = 100,000, uric acid = 8.5, BUN = 22, creatinine = 2. Appropriate interventions for the **PREVENTION** of tumor lysis syndrome would include all of the following **EXCEPT**
   A. fluid restriction <500 cc/day.
   B. aggressive IV hydration.
   C. initiation of allopurinol prior to treatment.
   D. diuresis.

42. Tumor lysis syndrome (TLS) is a complication of cancer therapy. TLS occurs most commonly in tumors that are
   A. large and rapidly dividing.
   B. slow growing and radiosensitive.
   C. slow growing and chemosensitive.
   D. small and rapidly dividing.

43. Individuals with the following cancers are at risk for developing increased intracranial pressure **EXCEPT** those with
   A. lung cancer.
   B. melanoma.
   C. breast cancer.
   D. multiple myeloma.

44. Systemic chemotherapy is *least* effective in which oncological emergency?
   A. Increased intracranial pressure.
   B. Superior vena cava syndrome.
   C. Cardiac tamponade.
   D. Spinal cord compression.

45. Which of the following signs/symptoms indicates increased intracranial pressure?
   A. Normal blood pressure.
   B. Agitation.
   C. Narrowing pulse pressure.
   D. Widening pulse pressure.

46. Which of the following interventions decreases the severity of symptoms associated with increased intracranial pressure?
   A. Instructing the patient to avoid the Valsalva maneuver.
   B. Keeping the patient supine.
   C Encouraging the patient to cough frequently.
   D. Administering furosemide.

47. Which mechanisms are responsible for an increase in intracranial pressure in patients with cancer?
   A. Tumor size and papilledema.
   B. Tumor type and peripheral edema.
   C. Tumor size and cerebral edema.
   D. Tumor type and grade.

48. One of the most common *immediate* symptoms of anaphylaxis is
   A. facial flushing.
   B. cyanosis of nail beds.
   C. development of bradycardia.
   D. decreased systolic blood pressure.

49. An indicator of the severity of an anaphylactic reaction is the
   A. amount of drug (or other allergen) given before the onset of symptoms.
   B. length of the interval between exposure and the onset of symptoms.
   C. history of previous allergic reactions.
   D. type of symptoms initially present.

40. *Answer:* **C**

 Rationale: The patient presents with a malignancy that has a high tumor burden and is on day two of his chemotherapy cycle. The chemotherapy is causing massive cell lysis, resulting in laboratory values and signs and symptoms consistent with tumor lysis syndrome.

41. *Answer:* **A**

 Rationale: Aggressive hydration, diuresis, and allopurinol are used in an attempt to maintain normal levels of potassium and uric acid.

42. *Answer:* **A**

 Rationale: Tumor lysis syndrome occurs most frequently in cancers with a rapidly growing large tumor burden after chemotherapy administration.

43. *Answer:* **D**

 Rationale: Tumor cells from breast cancer, lung cancer, and melanoma often metastasize to the brain.

44. *Answer:* **A**

 Rationale: Most chemotherapy drugs do not cross the blood–brain barrier to kill cancer cells. Chemotherapy has known efficacy, either alone or in combination with other treatment modalities, in superior vena cava syndrome, cardiac tamponade, and spinal cord compression.

45. *Answer:* **D**

 Rationale: Among the late signs of increased intracranial pressure are an increase in systolic blood pressure and a decrease in the diastolic blood pressure, which indicates a widening pulse pressure.

46. *Answer:* **A**

 Rationale: All responses except A cause increases in intracranial pressure and should not be encouraged.

47. *Answer:* **C**

 Rationale: The size of the tumor and the presence of cerebral edema compete for space within the skull, causing increased intracranial pressure.

48. *Answer:* **A**

 Rationale: This is the only immediate response; the others are late effects.

49. *Answer:* **D**

 Rationale: If the initial symptoms are of a respiratory nature, they are indicative of a much more severe anaphylactic reaction than the presence of flushing, itching, or hives.

50. Many of the chemotherapeutic agents that are used in the treatment of malignancy are capable of producing an anaphylactic reaction. A symptom of this reaction is
    A. bradycardia.
    B. laryngeal edema.
    C. decreased cardiac output.
    D. decreased urinary output.

51. Anaphylactic shock is a syndrome that is caused by which of the following?
    A. Decreased intravascular volume.
    B. Altered cellular metabolism.
    C. Loss of sympathetic tone to cardiovascular system.
    D. Exposure to a foreign antigen in a sensitized person.

52. While administering chemotherapeutic agents, nurses should be alert to the development of which of the following syndromes?
    A. Superior vena cava compression.
    B. Anaphylactic shock.
    C. Disseminated intravascular coagulopathy.
    D. Metabolic acidosis.

53. Mrs. S, a patient with recurrent ovarian carcinoma, has agreed to participate in a clinical trial involving a new agent with anaphylactic potential. What precautions should the nurse take the first time the drug is given?
    A. Premedicate the patient with diazepam.
    B. Reject the patient as a candidate for the study.
    C. Take vital signs prior to agent administration and every four hours thereafter.
    D. Administer the agent only in an environment where emergency drugs and equipment are readily available.

50. *Answer:* **B**

Rationale: Laryngeal edema is a symptom of an acute severe anaphylactic reaction.

51. *Answer:* **D**

Rationale: Anaphylactic shock associated with chemotherapy occurs secondary to an exposure to a foreign substance or antigen, which results in overstimulation of the immune system.

52. *Answer:* **B**

Rationale: While responses A, C, and D may occur in patients with metastatic malignancies, only B is a concern directly related to the administration of chemotherapy.

53. *Answer:* **D**

Rationale: Because an anaphylactic reaction may be a life-threatening emergency, appropriate emergency equipment and drugs should be readily available.

REFERENCES

Austin R, (1989). Management of Tumor Lysis Syndrome in the Ambulatory Setting. *Outpatient Chemotherapy.* 3 (1): 1–2, 9.

Barry SA, (1990). Septic Shock: Special Needs of Patients with Cancer. *Oncology Nursing Forum.* 16 (1): 31–35.

Chernecky CC, Ramsey PW, (1984). *Critical Nursing Care of the Client With Cancer.* Norwalk, CT: Appleton-Century-Crofts.

Dangel RB, (1991). Injury, Potential for, Related to Disseminated Intravascular Coagulopathy (DIC), in, McNally JC, Somerville CT, Miaskowski C, Rastad M, (eds). *Guidelines for Oncology Nursing Practice* (2nd ed). Philadelphia: WB Saunders. pp. 216–222.

Delaney TF, Oldfield EH, (1989). Spinal Cord Compression, in, DeVita VT, Hellman S, and Rosenberg S, (eds). *Cancer Principles and Practice of Oncology,* (3rd ed). Philadelphia: JB Lippincott, pp. 1980–1985.

Dietz K, Flaerty AM, (1990). Oncologic Emergencies, in, Groenwald SL, Frogge M, Goodman M, Yarbro CH, (eds). *Cancer Nursing Principles and Practice,* (2nd ed). Boston: Jones and Bartlett, pp. 652–655.

Elpern EH, (1990). Lung Cancer, in, Groenwald SL, Frogge MH, Goodman M, Yarbro CH, (eds). *Cancer Nursing Principles and Practice,* (2nd ed). Boston: Jones and Bartlett, pp. 951–973.

Finley JC, (1992). Nursing Care of Patients with Metabolic and Physiological Oncological Emergencies, in, Clark JC, McGee RF, (eds). *Core Curriculum for Oncology Nursing,* (2nd ed). Philadelphia: WB Saunders.

Gobel BH, (1990). Bleeding, in, Groenwald SL, Frogge MH, Goodman M, Yarbro CH, (eds). *Cancer Nursing Principles and Practice,* (2nd ed). Boston: Jones and Bartlett, pp. 467–484.

Gribbin ME, (1990). Could You Detect These Oncologic Emergencies? *RN.* 6(6): 37–41.

Hiller G, (1987). Cardiac Tamponade in the Oncology Patient. *Focus on Critical Care.* 14 (4): 32.

Hunter JC, (1992). Nursing Care of Patients with Structural Oncological Emergencies, in, Clark JC, McGee RF, (eds). *Core Curriculum for Oncology Nursing,* (2nd ed). Philadelphia: WB Saunders.

Lang-Kummer JL, (1990). Hypercalcemia, in, Groenwald SL, Frogge MH, Goodman M, Yarbro CH, (eds). *Cancer Nursing Principles and Practice,* (2nd ed). Boston: Jones and Bartlett, pp. 520–534.

McNally JC, Somerville ET, Miaskowski C, Rostad M, (eds), (1991). Circulation, in, *Guidelines for Oncology Nursing Practice,* (2nd ed). Philadelphia: WB Saunders. pp. 385–426.

Miaskowski C. (1991). Oncologic Emergencies, in, Baird SB, McCorkle R, Grant M, (eds). *Cancer Nursing A Comprehensive Textbook.* Philadelphia: W. B. Saunders Company, pp. 885–893.

Minna JD, Pass H, Glatstein E, Ihde D. (1989). Cancer of the Lung, in, DeVita VT, Hellman S, Rosenberg S, (eds). *Cancer Principles and Practice of Oncology,* (3rd ed). Philadelphia: JB Lippincott, pp. 591–705.

Morrison S, Shuey KM, (1990). Respiratory Dysfunction, in, Daeffler RJ, Petrosino BM (eds) *Manual of Oncology Nursing Practice.* Rockville, MD: Aspen Publishers, pp. 54–55.

Pass HI, (1989). Treatment of Malignant Pleural and Pericardial Effusion, in, DeVita VT, Hellman S, Rosenberg S, (eds). *Cancer Principles and Practice of Oncology,* (3rd ed). Philadelphia: JB Lippincott, pp. 2324–2335.

Poe D, Taylor LM, (1989). Syndrome of Inappropriate Antidiuretic Hormone: Assessment and Nursing Implications. *Oncology Nursing Forum* 16 (3): 373–381.

Valentine AS, Stewart JT, (1983). Oncologic Emergencies. *American Journal of Nursing.* 83 (9): 1283–1285.

Wegmann J, Hakius P, (1990). Central Nervous System Cancers, in, Groenwald SL, Frogge MH, Goodman M, Yarbro CH, (eds). *Cancer Nursing Principles and Practice,* (2nd ed). Boston: Jones and Bartlett, pp. 751–773.

Yahalom J, (1989), Superior Vena Cava Syndrome, in, DeVita VT, Hellman S, Rosenberg S, (eds). *Cancer Principles and Practice of Oncology,* (3rd ed). Philadelphia: JB Lippincott. pp. 1971–1977.

6
Issues and Trends in Cancer Care

Informed Consent, Legislation and Ethics
Toni Klatt-Ellis and Anne E. Belcher

Care Settings
Deborah Stephens Mills

Survivorship
Lois J. Loescher

Informed Consent, Legislation and Ethics
Toni Klatt-Ellis and Anne E. Belcher

Select the BEST answer for all of the following questions:

1. Ethics is primarily the study of
   A. how individuals should be allowed to die.
   B. what should be done in a given situation.
   C. what is lawful to do in light of cultural norms.
   D. why decisions are right or wrong.

2. Mr. L is a 52-year-old patient dying of colon cancer. He is divorced and has not seen his 12-year-old son for three years. He has asked the nursing staff not to release information about him to his ex-wife. Mr. L's ex-wife calls and explains that she has heard from friends that Mr. L is doing poorly. She wants to know his status because her son has told her that he really wants to see his dad before he dies. Ethically speaking, what is your **BEST** response to Mr. L's ex-wife's inquiries?
   A. Tell her about Mr. L's condition and ask her not to tell him how she got the information.
   B. Tell her about Mr. L's condition and then inform Mr. L and explain why you gave out information.
   C. Tell her you are sorry but you cannot give her any information about Mr. L's condition.
   D. Tell her to have the son come to the unit alone and that you will talk to him and let him see his dad.

1.   *Answer:* **B**

   Rationale: Ethics involves more than issues of dying. It is not a study of what is legal or lawful; there are no definite right or wrong answers. Ethics is the study of what *should* be done in situations regardless of laws, religious norms, or societal shortcomings.

2.   *Answer:* **C**

   Rationale: Unless the nurse talks with Mr. L and gets his permission, response C is the only ethical option. Mr. L has the right to decide who gets information and who does not.

3. Which one of the following is **TRUE** regarding ethical decision making in clinical situations?
   A. There is usually no one ethically correct answer to an ethical decision, but several equally ethical options based on the ethical model used.
   B. Ethics committees are best equipped to definitively recommend the correct ethical action in a given situation.
   C. Decisions made by knowledgeable health care professionals are usually more ethically correct than those made by family members.
   D. Lack of a clear-cut right or wrong ethical action results from inadequate assessment of the patient/family unit.

4. You would know your patient best understands the confidentiality provided in a clinical trial by the following statement he makes:
   A. "I know that although data about me may be published and presented, my name will not be used."
   B. "I know that no one will see the information gathered about me except the researchers."
   C. "I know that no one will be able to tell who I am from the data gathered about me."
   D. "I know that no one will be able to match my name to the data collected about me."

5. Which of the following actions does **NOT** fit within the nurse's role in informed consent?
   A. Withholding chemotherapy when a patient is confused and ambivalent about the proposed treatment plan and then notifying the physician.
   B. Initiating an explanation about the risks and benefits of a postoperative nursing procedure.
   C. Signing an informed consent when the legal guardian is not physically available to give permission to initiate chemotherapy treatments.
   D. Independently providing the patient with supplementary written educational material on postoperative side effects and their management.

6. Mr. S, a 32-year-old with leukemia, is deciding on whether he should enter a clinical trial. Mr. and Mrs. S are very close and have a very supportive relationship. Mrs. S has expressed what she thinks would be the best choice. Which one of the following actions by the nurse supports self-determination in this situation?
   A. Encourage Mrs. S to share her thoughts with her husband and offer yourself as a resource.
   B. Tell Mr. S what you think is best and then let him decide.
   C. Sit down with Mr. S and let him talk about the decision to be made.
   D. Encourage Mr. S to talk to someone else who has had to make a similar decision.

7. Mr. Z is a patient with advancing pancreatic cancer. He tells you he is going to make an appointment with his lawyer to have a living will drawn up. He expresses his wishes "not to be kept alive with IVs, tubes, and artificial things." You should keep the following in mind as you discuss Mr. Z's wishes with him:
   A. States vary in the degree to which they recognize living wills, and only a few allow withholding nutrition and hydration.
   B. Living wills are recognized and honored even though they may not be in writing on the chart.
   C. Ensuring that living wills are acknowledged is the responsibility of the patient's physician.
   D. According to definitions of "mentally competent," patients in an advanced disease state cannot initiate a living will document.

3. *Answer:* **A**

Rationale: Ethical decisions rarely have one right or wrong answer, but several equally attractive courses of action. Depending on the ethical model used, different conclusions may be reached. Family input helps guide decisions to a more satisfactory ethical end. Hospital ethics committees vary in composition and purpose and may not be the best decision-making body for ethical issues.

4. *Answer:* **A**

Rationale: In a clinical trial, data collectors and nurses may see information gathered about a patient. Additionally, B implies that no journal publication or professional presentations can be done. Responses C and D speak to anonymity, not confidentiality.

5. *Answer:* **C**

Rationale: Independent actions in giving information about any side effects, management of side effects, and nursing procedures are within nursing's scope of practice. Signing a consent form is not within any health care professional's scope of practice.

6. *Answer:* **C**

Rationale: Only response C supports Mr. S in making a decision that is best for him, without intentional interference by another.

7. *Answer:* **A**

Rationale: The laws on living wills state they must be in writing and signed by the patient. Furthermore, it is the hospital's responsibility to ascertain if a living will exists and inform patients of their rights regarding a living will. Patients with advancing, progressive, and/or terminal disease can have a living will drawn up if they are still fully mentally intact. States do vary in recognition of living will documents and how extensive and specific they can be.

8.   Mr. Z is a patient with advancing pancreatic cancer. You have been discussing his rights regarding living wills. Mr. Z tells you, "I don't want to be kept alive with IVs, tubes, and artificial things when it comes time to go." Which one of the following statements indicates to you that Mr. Z understands his rights regarding living wills?

   A.   "I feel comfortable knowing that I will be allowed to die without the discomfort of any feeding tubes and IVs."
   B.   "I am reassured knowing that I don't have to express my wishes in writing in case I change my mind at the last minute."
   C.   "I am concerned that if I have a living will done now, without a mental health evaluation, it will not be valid."
   D.   "I know that if I have a living will document drawn up, chances are good that I will be able to control the conditions under which my care is provided."

9.   The next **two** questions relate to the following scenario: Mr. B has terminal head and neck cancer. He is unresponsive. Mr. B is a widower and has no children. He has been on a morphine drip for two months. The nursing staff have been titrating the morphine drip as needed for pain control. Nurses consistently report that Mr. B seems to be comfortable. Mr. B's physician makes rounds every day and seems to be very uncomfortable in Mr. B's room. Every day Mr. B's physician spends less and less time in his rounds with Mr. B. For the past three days, the physician has written an order to increase the morphine drip by 10–15 mg/hr each day. Today you make rounds with the doctor and he asks you about Mr. B's pain control. You tell the doctor that you think Mr. B is comfortable. Later you notice that the physician wrote an order to increase the morphine drip by 20 mg/hr. Of the following, which one is the *most critical* ethical question that must be resolved?

   A.   Should the nurses be the ones to titrate the morphine drip for pain control?
   B.   Was it ethical to increase Mr. B's morphine drip by 10–15 mg/hr for the past three days?
   C.   What is the physician's intent in increasing the morphine drip rate?
   D.   Should the nurse follow the physician's order to increase the morphine drip?

8.   *Answer:* **D**

Rationale: Living wills do not assure that individuals can control whether nutrition and hydration are provided. Response A indicates that Mr. Z may not fully understand this. Living wills must be in writing to be valid. If an individual changes his wishes, documentation of this in the chart is legally binding. Response C indicates a misunderstanding of the definition of "mentally competent." Response D is correct because living wills cannot "promise" that a patient's wishes will be fully implemented; however, living wills certainly increase an individual's "chances of control" over the way in which terminal care is carried out.

9.   *Answer:* **D**

Rationale: Response D is correct because it is the question that must be resolved to decide on the next action to take. Information addressing the question raised in response C will be helpful in resolving the question presented in response D. Response D, however, is the most critical question that must be resolved.

10.   Using a utilitarian-based ethical decision-making model, which one of the following actions is most appropriate in the case of Mr. B?

    A.   Call the physician to determine his intent in increasing the rate and tell him you feel it is wrong to turn up the drip rate.

    B.   Take a poll on the unit, by secret ballot, and implement the action that the majority of the nurses reason is appropriate.

    C.   Decide which ethical principles are most important in this situation, rank them in order of importance, and then take the action that is congruent with the highest-ranked ethical principle.

    D.   Reason what possible outcomes would likely be produced by each possible course of action. Take the action that seems likely to produce the best outcome.

11.   Mrs. X has been diagnosed with primary bone cancer and chemotherapy has been ordered. You are preparing to go into Mrs. X's room to administer chemotherapy when her two daughters approach you and ask you not to talk with Mrs. X about any side effects of the drugs. Mrs. X's daughters fear that their mother will refuse to take chemotherapy treatments if she knows she may get sick or lose her hair. In deciding how to respond to this situation, you should keep in mind which one of the following statements about patients' rights and informed consent?

    A.   States differ in the amount of freedom given to family members to make decisions regarding disclosure of information.

    B.   National laws allow for withholding information if treatment is vitally needed and disclosing information will delay initiation of treatment.

    C.   A patient does not have to be informed of all possible risks and benefits of treatment if informed consent can be obtained from competent immediate family members.

    D.   Fear that a patient will refuse treatment when informed about risks is not a sufficient reason to withhold information.

12.   When talking with a legislator about tobacco control, which one of the following statements would likely have the most impact?

    A.   National statistics show that 35% of individuals alive today smoke and 65% of them will some day die of lung cancer.

    B.   Studies show that most tobacco users start using tobacco in their teens and advertising and availability are two strong influences in initiation of tobacco use.

    C.   National data indicate that Southern states have more of a problem with tobacco addiction and tobacco-induced health problems per capita than do the states in the North.

    D.   Study data indicate that the health status of potentially up to 80%–90% of your constituency are affected negatively by either first-hand or second-hand smoke.

10.   *Answer:* **D**

Rationale: Response D uses utilitarian reasoning to resolve an ethical question and to decide on an appropriate action. Response C is the deontological approach. Responses A and B follow no ethical model of decision making.

11.   *Answer:* **D**

Rationale: National and/or state laws do not set parameters for information that may be withheld from individuals. Here, the issue is not a legal one. The focus should be what should Mrs. X be told. Informed consent for treatment can only be given by a competent person receiving the treatment. Patients have a right to an explanation of all risks and benefits of treatment and to refuse treatment if they so choose.

12.   *Answer:* **B**

Rationale: The three incorrect responses (A, C, D) may be alarming information and may help to define the impact tobacco use is having on society. However, only response B provides the legislator with information that specifically addresses controlling the initiation of tobacco use. It gives specific direction for the content of a legislative bill. It is the kind of information that motivates legislators to action.

13. Which one of the following pieces of legislation is aimed at improving the potential for rehabilitation and full recovery from cancer? Legislation which
   A. requires surgeons to explain to women with breast cancer all treatment options.
   B. prevents an individual from losing insurance for three months after resignation from a job, even if they are diagnosed with cancer during that three months.
   C. requires insurance companies to fully reimburse for the cost of an annual Pap smear and mammogram.
   D. provides Medicare and Medicaid reimbursement for physical therapy for hospice patients.

14. Which one of the following is an example of cancer prevention legislation?
   A. A bill to increase the amount Medicare will reimburse for an annual Pap smear.
   B. A bill to provide Medicare coverage for biannual screening mammography.
   C. A bill that limits tobacco advertising at sports events.
   D. A bill that requires physicians to inform patients over the age of fifty of the American Cancer Society's guidelines for cancer checkups.

15. Mr. Z is a 62-year-old patient with lymphoma who is expressing difficulty in getting his insurance to cover the cost of chemotherapy treatments. Your **BEST** response to him, based on your knowledge of current regulations for off-label use of drugs, is:
   A. "Be sure to tell the physician's office of the difficulty you are having so that a letter of explanation can be sent about your treatment."
   B. "Insurance may not reimburse for the cost of drugs used to treat cancers when this was not part of the original approved use for the drug."
   C. "Call your insurance representative and explain your difficulty in getting reimbursed when generic drugs are used."
   D. "Ask your physician to consider writing a prescription for the drugs so that you can bring the drugs to the clinic when you get a treatment."

16. Mrs. L, a 67-year-old patient, has alopecia from chemotherapy treatments. She is living on a very limited Social Security income and is concerned about the cost of a wig. Your **BEST** response to her questions regarding reimbursement for hairpieces for alopecia caused by cancer treatment is:
   A. "Medicare reimburses for the cost of wigs."
   B. "Medicare reimburses for wig expense up to a certain amount, and then supplemental insurance covers the remainder."
   C. "Medicare reimburses for wigs if a minimum deductible has been met."
   D. "Medicare does not reimburse the expense of a wig, but some private insurance carriers do."

13. *Answer:* **A**

Rationale: Responses B and C are not addressing rehabilitation; they are addressing treatment and early detection. Response D is addressing an aspect of rehabilitation; however, hospice patients are not expected to fully recover. Response A allows a woman to know that, for stage I breast disease, a lumpectomy and radiation is as effective as mastectomy. Full recovery and rehabilitation potential are much better with lumpectomy and radiation. Legislation has been proposed, but not yet passed, to address the problem of women not receiving an explanation of treatment options.

14. *Answer:* **C**

Rationale: Although all have been actual proposed legislation, C is the only option that addresses prevention. A, B, and D are involved with early detection.

15. *Answer:* **B**

Rationale: Sometimes using a drug for a nonapproved cancer treatment (one that is not listed on the label of the drug information) will be considered "experimental" by some insurance carriers, and they will not pay for the treatment. This occurs despite extensive research showing that the drug is appropriate for this treatment use.

16. *Answer:* **D**

Rationale: Legislation has not been passed to authorize Medicare reimbursement for wigs needed because of alopecia from cancer treatment. Some private insurance carriers, however, consider it as a rehabilitation measure and cover it under specific clauses in policies.

REFERENCES

Donovan CT, (1990). Ethics in Cancer Nursing Practice, in, Groenwald SL, Frogge MH, Goodman M, Yarbro CH, (eds). *Cancer Nursing Principles and Practice*, (2nd ed). Boston: Jones and Bartlett, pp. 1201–1215.

———— (1986). Ethics and Cancer. *CA* 36 (2). Atlanta, GA: American Cancer Society.

Chamorro T, (1991). Legal Responsibilities of the Nurse, in, Baird SB, McCorkle R, Grant M, (eds). *Cancer Nursing A Comprehensive Textbook*. Philadelphia: W. B. Saunders Company, pp. 1139–1148.

Francoeur RT, (1983). *Biomedical Ethics*. New York: John Wiley and Sons.

Fry ST, (1991). Ethics in Cancer Care, in, Baird SB, McCorkle R, Grant M, (eds). *Cancer Nursing A Comprehensive Textbook*. Philadelphia: W. B. Saunders Company, pp. 31–37.

Gevin RR, Richters JC, (1992). Selected Ethical Issues in Cancer Care, in, Clark JC, McGee RF, (eds). *Core Curriculum for Oncology Nursing*, (2nd ed). Philadelphia: WB Saunders.

Gullatte MM, (1992). Legal Issues Influencing Cancer Care, in, Clark JC, McGee RF, (eds). *Core Curriculum for Oncology Nursing*, (2nd ed). Philadelphia: WB Saunders.

Levine ME, (1982). Bioethics of Cancer Nursing. *Rehabilitation Nursing*. March–April: 27–30, 47.

Lisson EL, (1989). Ethics and Pain Management. *Seminars in Oncology Nursing*. 5 (2): 114–119.

Neil EA, (1987). Treatment Decisions with the Terminally Ill Incompetent Patient. *Nursing Economics*. 5 (1): 32–35.

Schoene-Siefert B, Childress JF, (1986). How Much Should the Cancer Patient Know and Decide? *Cancer*. 36 (2): 85–94.

Wegmann J, Jassak P, (eds), (1989). Ethical Issues in Cancer Care. Seminars in Oncology Nursing. 5(2): 75–131.

Care Settings

Deborah Stephens Mills

Select the BEST answer for all of the following questions:

1. In determining the need for an oncology unit, the principle variable to be considered is
    A. the availability of nurses skilled in cancer care.
    B. the cost of organizing a specialty unit.
    C. the percentage of cancer admissions to the hospital.
    D. the support of attending physicians and area oncologists.

2. The most effective intervention that a home care nurse uses is
    A. providing twenty-four-hour on-call availability.
    B. collaborating with primary physicians.
    C. teaching the proper use of prn medications.
    D. supporting the primary caregiver(s).

3. The National Coalition of Cancer Survivors (NCCS) promotes a special event each year. This is
    A. "Celebrate Life."
    B. the "Great American Smokeout."
    C. the "Humor Project."
    D. "We Can" Weekend.

4. Patients and families contract with a cancer nurse in private practice
    A. only on the recommendation of their physician.
    B. to obtain a second opinion on cancer therapy.
    C. to negotiate a job discrimination suit.
    D. for specialized education and counseling.

5. Appliance fitting and teaching a patient to care for his colostomy postoperatively are nursing activities that are considered
    A. preventive.
    B. restorative.
    C. supportive.
    D. palliative

6. "To improve the quality of life for maximum productivity with minimum dependence, regardless of life expectancy" is the goal of
    A. survivor advocacy.
    B. cancer nursing.
    C. cancer rehabilitation.
    D. hospice nursing.

7. The hospice care setting that relies on the home as the place of care is a
    A. community-based program.
    B. hospital-based program.
    C. associated oncology practice.
    D. free-standing hospice.

8. Hospice is a concept of care that concentrates on rehumanizing the experience of dying by
    A. focusing on the family's need of continued support beyond the patient's death.
    B. joining optimal symptom control with sensitive, noninvasive caring.
    C. allowing all patients to die in the comfort of their homes.
    D. providing respectful and dignified care with the help of friends and volunteers.

9. If given the choice, the preferred care setting of most patients is
    A. ambulatory care.
    B. in-patient oncology unit.
    C. in-patient general med-surg unit.
    D. major referral center.

1. *Answer:* **C**

   Rationale: Development of an oncology unit should occur only if there is a population to use the services.

2. *Answer:* **D**

   Rationale: By supporting the primary caregivers, the nurse may prolong and enhance the experience of care in the home.

3. *Answer:* **A**

   Rationale: "Celebrate Life" day is the annual event sponsored by the NCCS to celebrate survivorship.

4. *Answer:* **D**

   Rationale: Education of patients and families and counseling are functions of the nurse within nurse practice acts.

5. *Answer:* **B**

   Rationale: These activities promote self-care and rehabilitation and, hence, are restorative in nature.

6. *Answer:* **C**

   Rationale: This statement describes ONS's position on cancer rehabilitation.

7. *Answer:* **A**

   Rationale: Community-based hospices mostly rely on volunteer staff to support patients and families in the home.

8. *Answer:* **B**

   Rationale: The philosophy of hospice promotes palliation and support as opposed to therapeutic, cure-oriented goals.

9. *Answer:* **A**

   Rationale: Most patients prefer to remain at home whenever possible even if it means daily visits to an ambulatory care setting.

REFERENCES

Amenta MO, (1984). Hospice USA 1984—Steadying and Holding. *Oncology Nursing Forum.* 11 (5): 68–74.

Amenta M, (1991). Hospice Services, in, Baird SB, McCorkle R, Grant M, (eds). *Cancer Nursing A Comprehensive Textbook.* Philadelphia: W. B. Saunders Company, pp. 1033–1043.

Anderson JL, (1989). The Nurses' Role in Cancer Rehabilitation. *Cancer Nursing.* 12 (2): 85–94.

Baigis-Smith J, Hagopian GA, (1991). Community Assessment: Congruence of Needs and Resources, in, Baird SB, McCorkle R, Grant M, (eds). *Cancer Nursing A Comprehensive Textbook.* Philadelphia: W. B. Saunders Company, pp. 1044–1056.

Balnk JJ, et al, (1989). Perceived Home Care Needs of Cancer Patients and their Caregivers. *Cancer Nursing.* 12 (2): 78–84.

Brown JK, (1985). Ambulatory Services: The Mainstay of Cancer Nursing Care. *Oncology Nursing Forum.* 12 (1): 57–59.

Dudas S, Carlson CE, (1988). Cancer Rehabilitation. *Oncology Nursing Forum.* 15 (2): 183–188.

Farley BA, (1991). Ambulatory Care Services, in, Baird SB, McCorkle R, Grant M, (eds). *Cancer Nursing A Comprehensive Textbook.* Philadelphia: W. B. Saunders Company, pp. 1011–1022.

Gambosi JR, Ulreich S, (1990). Recovering From Cancer: A Nursing Intervention Program Recognizing Survivorship. *Oncology Nursing Forum.* 17 (2): 215–219.

Grady C, (1989). Acquired Immunodeficiency Syndrome: The Impact on Professional Nursing Practice. *Cancer Nursing.* 12 (1): 1–9.

Harris MD, Parente CA, (1991). Home Care Services, in, Baird SB, McCorkle R, Grant M, (eds). *Cancer Nursing A Comprehensive Textbook.* Philadelphia: W. B. Saunders Company, pp. 1023–1032.

Lewis FM, (1990). Strengthening Family Support. *Cancer.* 65 : 952–959.

Mills DS, (1992). Changes in Oncology Health Care Settings, in, Clark JC, McGee RF, (eds). *Core Curriculum for Oncology Nursing,* (2nd ed). Philadelphia: WB Saunders.

Moinpour CM, Polissar L, (1989). Factors Affecting Place of Death of Hospice and Non-hospice Cancer Patients. *American Journal of Public Health.* 79 (11) : 1549–1551.

Mosely JR, Brown JS, (1985). The Organization and Operation of Oncology Units. *Oncology Nursing Forum.* 12 (5) : 17–24.

McCorkle R, et al., (1979). A New Beginning: The Opening of a Multidisciplinary Cancer Unit. *Cancer Nursing,* Part I. 2 (3) : 201–209. Part II : 2 (4) : 269–278.

McMahon KM, Coyne N, (1989). Symptom Management in Patients with AIDS. *Seminars in Oncology Nursing.* 5 (4) : 289–301.

Padilla G, Kirshner T, (1991). Continuity of Care and Discharge Planning, in, Baird SB, McCorkle R, Grant M, (eds). *Cancer Nursing A Comprehensive Textbook.* Philadelphia: W. B. Saunders Company, pp. 1000–1010.

Rose MA, (1989). Health Promotion and Risk Prevention: Applications for Cancer Survivors. *Oncology Nursing Forum.* 16 (3) : 335–340.

Smith SN, Bohnet N, (1983). Organization and Administration of Hospice Care. *Journal of Nursing Administration.* 13 (11) : 10–16.

Watson PB, (1990). Cancer Rehabilitation: The Evolution of a Concept. *Cancer Nursing.* 13 (1) : 2–12.

Wright P, Dyck S, (1984). Expressed Concerns of Adult Cancer Patients' Family Members. *Cancer Nursing.* 7 (10) : 371–374.

Yates JW, Lyons C, (1991). The Organization of Cancer Service Settings, in, Baird SB, McCorkle R, Grant M, (eds). *Cancer Nursing A Comprehensive Textbook.* Philadelphia: W. B. Saunders Company, pp. 993–999.

Survivorship

Lois J. Loescher

Select the BEST answer for all of the following questions:

1. Which of the following resources is available on a national level for cancer survivors experiencing employment discrimination?
   A. The National Coalition for Cancer Survivorship (NCCS).
   B. The Rehabilitation Act of 1973.
   C. The Employees' Retirement and Income Security Act (ERISA).
   D. All of the above.

2. Certain steps should be taken by cancer survivors who are the targets of discrimination by employers. What is the next step to be taken after contacting the legal counsel at the place of employment to discuss how the Rehabilitation Act of 1973 affects them?
   A. Contact their U.S. congressional representative to confront the employer about the discrimination.
   B. Consult with an attorney specializing in employment law.
   C. Contact the State Department of Labor, Civil Rights Division, for further assistance.
   D. Contact the State Insurance Department, Employment Division, for further assistance.

3. Laws that protect cancer survivors against employment discrimination when they are qualified for their jobs
   A. are the same laws that protect the mentally or physically disabled.
   B. are only legislated through state governments.
   C. only apply to private employers.
   D. are currently nonexistent.

4. Which one of the following descriptions about insurance is **NOT** true?
   A. New applications for insurance can never be legally refused.
   B. If the survivor had a policy before the diagnosis of cancer, that policy can be canceled by insurers following a cancer diagnosis.
   C. Insurance companies may reduce existing benefits of a policy after a cancer diagnosis.
   D. Insurance policies for survivors cost more and take longer to obtain.

5. A serious consequence of cancer therapy is the development of second malignancies. All of the following statements about second malignancies are true **EXCEPT**
   A. treatment-related second malignancies are frequently fatal.
   B. second malignancies account for only a small portion of mortality in long-term survivors.
   C. some second malignancies occur by chance alone.
   D. most second malignancies will occur within five years of treatment.

6. The care and rehabilitation of cancer survivors should include strategies to promote which one of the following behaviors?
   A. Cancer prevention and early detection.
   B. Encouraging family members who are at high risk for cancers to receive counseling and care.
   C. Reducing risk factors for other diseases.
   D. All of the above.

1. *Answer:* **A**

   Rationale: The federal Americans with Disabilities Act, effective in 1992, balances the Federal Rehabilitation Act of 1973 by covering individuals who are working for, or desire to work for, private employers.

2. *Answer:* **B**

   Rationale: Although the Federal Rehabilitation Act of 1973 is limited to those employers who receive federal funding, it can offer protection to those who qualify and feel discriminated against because of a real or perceived (by the employer) handicap.

3. *Answer:* **A**

   Rationale: In general, discrimination against cancer survivors who are qualified for jobs, but are treated differently solely because of their cancer history, violates most laws that prohibit discrimination against the handicapped.

4. *Answer:* **A**

   Rationale: The availability of adequate health insurance is rarely guaranteed, and the problems created when attempting to secure or obtain these benefits can be financially and emotionally devastating.

5. *Answer:* **D**

   Rationale: Some second malignancies will occur by chance alone. Others may occur because first and second cancers share common etiologies (i.e., smoking). Some second tumors occur because of a genetic predisposition to developing second cancers (i.e., sarcomas following retinoblastoma), and some may be related to the treatment of the first cancer. Second malignancies are a late sequela of cancer therapy.

6. *Answer:* **D**

   Rationale: The nurse's role in cancer rehabilitation should include strategies to promote new behaviors for enhancing the early detection of recurrent disease and reducing risk factors for second malignancies, along with other diseases that could be prevented by diet, exercise, and smoking cessation.

7. Obstacles to cancer rehabilitation include
   A. philosophy and attitudes of health care professionals differ from those held by the public.
   B. lack of coordinated interdisciplinary care and lack of adequate reimbursement for rehabilitation services.
   C. little research supporting the efficacy of rehabilitation interventions and difficulty in obtaining funding for cancer rehabilitation research.
   D. all of the above.

8. Cancer survivors are often confronted with all of the following spiritual/existential issues **EXCEPT**
   A. changes in life priorities after critical evaluation and a search for meaning in life.
   B. altered socioeconomic status.
   C. a new passion for life.
   D. a greater self-love or self-acceptance.

9. When survivors who are doing well see others with cancer who are not doing as well, they may experience
   A. survivor guilt.
   B. waiting room phenomenon.
   C. ultra-altruism.
   D. euphoria.

10. Nursing interventions for the acute survival stage include all of the following **EXCEPT**
   A. providing measures to allay anxiety and fears about death.
   B. assessing survivor and family needs and coping skills.
   C. encouraging regular follow-up examinations.
   D. exit interviews as patients complete their initial course of therapy.

11. A comprehensive interdisciplinary long-term follow-up program for cancer survivors would most benefit survivors in which stage?
   A. The acute survival stage.
   B. The extended survival stage.
   C. The permanent survival stage.
   D. All of the above stages.

12. Nursing interventions to assist the survivor in dealing with fears of recurrence are most applicable in which survival stage?
   A. The acute stage.
   B. The extended stage.
   C. The permanent stage.
   D. All of the above stages.

13. Rehabilitation of cancer survivors should ideally begin
   A. at the time of diagnosis.
   B. once treatment is determined.
   C. after treatment is finished.
   D. when the survivor has no evidence of disease.

14. Which statement best describes the cancer survivor's fears of recurrence and death?
   A. These fears are most prevalent during diagnosis and initial treatment of cancer.
   B. These fears usually begin to subside two to three years after completion of therapy.
   C. Sometimes these fears persist many years after completion of therapy.
   D. All of the above statements describe the cancer survivor's fears of recurrence and death.

15. Primary factors contributing to the potential development of long-term and late effects are
   A. the type, location, size, and extent of the primary tumor.
   B. the type and aggressiveness of therapy.
   C. the age and health status of the individual at the time of diagnosis.
   D. all of the above.

16. Cancer survivors who have received radiation to the head and neck are at risk for
   A. serious or fatal strokes.
   B. sensory loss.
   C. leukoencephalopathy.
   D. all of the above.

7. *Answer:* **D**

    Rationale: Issues of survivorship are of increased concern to health care professionals. Focus should be broadened beyond the prevention, early detection, and treatment measures to include the structure, process, and outcome of rehabilitation care. Obstacles to rehabilitation must be recognized and overcome for rehabilitation to occur.

8. *Answer:* **B**

    Rationale: Living through a life-threatening experience heightens the desire to get on with living and personally evaluate life's priorities and meaning.

9. *Answer:* **A**

    Rationale: Comparisons may be made with another patient, causing survivors to wonder, "Why am I doing well and they aren't?" Similar to questions arising around the time of initial diagnosis, attempts to justify "why me" or "why not me" may resurface. Hence the survivor's ongoing involvement with follow-up care is characterized by mixed emotional reactions and multiple concerns.

10. *Answer:* **C**

    Rationale: Expert coaching is based on knowledge of both the disease and the treatments and their relationship. Follow-up examinations are addressed in the extended and permanent stages.

11. *Answer:* **C**

    Rationale: Health care practitioners have an obligation to participate in the development and implementation of interventions that maximize rehabilitation after treatment.

12. *Answer:* **B**

    Rationale: The season of extended survival is dominated by fear of recurrence.

13. *Answer:* **A**

    Rationale: The cancer experience is a continuum. Comprehensive rehabilitation involves addressing issues at each stage.

14. *Answer:* **D**

    Rationale: In a review of the literature, death anxiety is greater in survivors within two years of therapy as compared to those with more protracted survival. However, some have found that these fears are more common during active treatment, but may persist years after therapy is completed.

15. *Answer:* **D**

    Rationale: The occurrence, frequency, and severity of long-term and late sequelae depend on all of the listed factors.

16. *Answer:* **D**

    Rationale: Acute or chronic toxic radiotherapy can lead to long-term or late neurovascular problems in cancer survivors.

17. Effects that occur chronically after cessation of therapy are usually called
    A. progressive effects.
    B. long-term effects.
    C. iatrogenic effects.
    D. all of the above.

18. According to Mullan's "seasons of survival," when is the survivor usually referred to as a patient?
    A. During the extended stage.
    B. During the acute stage.
    C. During the permanent stage.
    D. All of the above.

19. Which one of the following statements **BEST** characterizes a person in the *permanent* stage of survival?
    A. The survivor's cancer status has gradually evolved to where the probability for disease recurrence is minimal.
    B. The survivor is cancer-free.
    C. The survivor has reached the five-year disease-free mark after completing therapy.
    D. All of the above statements characterize a permanent survivor.

20. Persons in the *extended* stage of survival are
    A. finished with all medical treatments.
    B. in remission or on maintenance therapy.
    C. in the final stages of life.
    D. undergoing initial therapy.

21. Which statement best describes the acute survival stage? The acute stage begins at the moment of diagnosis and
    A. extends through completion of treatment.
    B. extends through the initial treatment.
    C. ends before treatment starts.
    D. ends when there is no evidence of disease.

22. Six million Americans alive today have a history of cancer. How many of these are considered cancer "survivors"?
    A. All six million.
    B. The three million who are disease-free.
    C. Anyone who has completed treatment.
    D. The two million who have not had recurrence of disease.

23. A recent and more comprehensive definition of a cancer survivor is
    A. a person with a history of cancer.
    B. a family member or significant other who survives a loved one who died from cancer.
    C. one who is alive five years after cancer diagnosis and/or therapy.
    D. all of the above.

24. Cancer survivors have traditionally been defined as individuals who
    A. have no evidence of disease when cancer treatment ends.
    B. relapse and then go into remission for prolonged periods.
    C. are alive five years after cancer diagnosis and/or therapy.
    D. all of the above.

17. *Answer:* **B**

Rationale: Long-term effects of cancer and cancer therapy begin during the acute or extended stages and continue indefinitely after treatment ends.

18. *Answer:* **B**

Rationale: The acute stage is a medically oriented stage.

19. *Answer:* **A**

Rationale: This stage is roughly equated with the phenomenon called "cure." Permanent survival has several dimensions beyond those of victory over the disease, specifically a kinship and continuum with the previous seasons of survival. There is no moment of cure, but rather an evolution from the phase of extended survival into a period where the activity of the disease, or the likelihood of its return, is sufficiently small that the cancer can be considered permanently arrested.

20. *Answer:* **B**

Rationale: When the survivor goes into remission or has terminated the basic, rigorous course of treatment, the extended stage has begun. This stage is dominated by fear of recurrence, physical limitations, and adapting to a "healthy" world.

21. *Answer:* **B**

Rationale: The acute stage is really the medical stage and is dominated by diagnosis and therapeutic efforts to stem the tide of illness. Fear and anxiety are constant elements of this stage, which can create a mental state of ill-being that is often more difficult to deal with than the cancer itself. Pain may be present, along with side effects of treatments. The survivor's family is often overlooked in the acute stage.

22. *Answer:* **A**

Rationale: Everyone with a cancer history is a cancer survivor.

23. *Answer:* **A**

Rationale: Survival is generic and applies to everyone diagnosed with cancer, regardless of the course of the illness. Survival begins at the time of diagnosis and ends at death.

24. *Answer:* **C**

Rationale: Cancer survivors have historically been labelled as cured if no evidence of cancer exists after five years, without much reference to surviving throughout treatment.

REFERENCES

Crother H, (1987). Health Insurance: Problems and Solutions For People With Cancer Histories. *Proceedings of the 5th National Conference on Human Values and Cancer*. San Francisco: American Cancer Society, pp. 100–109.

Dow KH, (1990). The Enduring Seasons in Survival. *Oncology Nursing Forum*. 17 : 511–516.

Dudas S, Carlson CE, (1988). Cancer Rehabilitation. *Oncology Nursing Forum*. 15 : 183–188.

Fraser MC, Tucker MA, (1989). Second Malignancies Following Cancer Therapy. *Seminars in Oncology Nursing*. 5 : 43–55.

Hoffman B, (1989). Current Issues of Cancer Survivorship. *Oncology*. 3 : 85–88.

Hoffman B, (1989). Cancer Survivors at Work: Job Problems and Illegal Discrimination. *Oncology Nursing Forum*. 16 : 39–43.

Leigh S, (1992). Cancer Survivorship Issues, in, Clark JC, McGee RF, (eds). *Core Curriculum for Oncology Nursing*, (2nd ed). Philadelphia: WB Saunders.

Li FP, (1985). Second Cancers, in, DeVita VT, Hellman S, Rosenberg S, (eds). *Cancer Principles and Practice of Oncology*, (2nd ed). Philadelphia: JB Lippincott, pp. 2042–2049.

Loescher LJ, Welch-McCaffrey D, Leigh SA, et al., (1989). Surviving Adult Cancers (Part I): Physiological Effects. *Annals of Internal Medicine*. 111 : 411–432.

Loescher LJ, Clark L, Atweel JR, et al., (1990). The Impact of the Cancer Experience on Long-term Survivors. *Oncology Nursing Forum*. 17 : 223–229.

McNally JC, Somerville ET, Miaskowski C, Rastad M, (eds). (1991). Sexuality, in, *Guidelines for Oncology Nursing Practice*, (2nd ed). Philadelphia: WB Saunders, pp. 337–350.

Mullan F, (1984). Re-Entry: The Educational Needs of the Cancer Survivor. *Health Education Quarterly*. (Supp) 10 : 88–94.

Mullan F, (1985). Seasons of Survival: Reflections of a Physician With Cancer. *New England Journal of Medicine*. 313 : 270–273.

Mullan F, Hoffman B, and the Editors of Consumers Reports Books (eds), (1990). *An Almanac of Practical Resources for Cancer Survivors: Charting the Journey*. Consumers Union, NY: Mount Vernon.

Mayer D, O'Connor L, (1989). Rehabilitation of Persons with Cancer: An ONS Position Statement. *Oncology Nursing Forum*. 16 : 433.

Rose MA, (1989). Health Promotion and Risk Prevention: Applications for Cancer Survivors. *Oncology Nursing Forum*. 16 : 335–340.

Welch-McCaffrey D, Hoffman B, Leigh S, Loescher LJ, (1989). Surviving Adult Cancers (Part II): Psychosocial Implications. *Annals of Internal Medicine*. 111 : 517–524.

Welch-McCaffrey D, Leigh S, Loescher LJ, Hoffman B, (1990). Psychosocial Dimensions: Issues in Survivorship, in, Groenwald SL, Frogge MH, Goodman M, Yarbro CH, (eds). *Cancer Nursing Principles and Practice*, (2nd ed). Boston: Jones and Bartlett, pp. 373–382.

7
Professional Issues

Mary Cunningham and Linda Leah Hunter

Select the BEST answer for all of the following questions:

1. Which one of the following statements regarding stress is **INCORRECT**?
   A. Stress is necessary for life.
   B. Individual judgment and evaluation of the stimulus influences perception of the stimulus but not the nature of the response.
   C. Stress becomes a problem when the level of stress exceeds one's ability to effectively respond.
   D. Professional stress demands adaptation in the performance of one's professional role.

2. Characteristics of a nurse that contribute to stress and/or burnout include all of the following **EXCEPT**
   A. strong dependency needs.
   B. lack of identification with patients and families.
   C. overdedication and overcommitment.
   D. diffuse ego boundaries.

3. Stress demands adaptational change. Which of the following responses is a manifestation of stress?
   A. Repetitive accidents, constant state of fatigue, and sleep disturbances.
   B. Excessive concentration.
   C. Detachment from responsibility for others.
   D. Compassion and understanding.

4. A strategy for self-management of stress may include
   A. isolating oneself from the situation.
   B. fostering a competitive work environment.
   C. establishing realistic goals and self-expectations.
   D. concentrating on work-related topics.

5. A right of the nurse in the workplace is to
   A. refuse if substantiated with cause.
   B. influence scheduling.
   C. be treated with respect.
   D. determine assignments.

The statements in questions 6–10 jeopardize characteristics that are necessary for the development of the professional and the fulfillment of a profession. Select the characteristic of the profession that is compromised by each statement.

6. There is a lack of consensus regarding uniform preparation of nurses for entry into practice.
   A. Authority.
   B. Autonomy.
   C. Commitment.
   D. Specialized knowledge.

7. There is a lack of monetary rewards for experienced nurses; career advancement opportunities for clinicians are only into management positions.
   A. Authority.
   B. Autonomy.
   C. Vital service.
   D. Commitment.

1. *Answer:* **B**

   Rationale: Lazarus views stress as a transaction between an individual and the environment. The individual is the focal mediator between the stress stimulus and the response. Individual judgment and evaluation of the stimulus influence perception of the stimulus as well as the nature of the response.

2. *Answer:* **B**

   Rationale: Overidentification with patients and families is a characteristic that increases an individual's vulnerability to stress and the development of burnout.

3. *Answer:* **A**

   Rationale: Stress responses and adaptational changes are physical, intellectual, and emotional in nature.

4. *Answer:* **C**

   Rationale: Collaborative relationships, not competitive relationships, are conducive to positive stress.

5. *Answer:* **A**

   Rationale: Nurses have the right to refuse without making excuses or feeling guilty.

6. *Answer:* **D**

   Rationale: Specialized knowledge implies that professional practice is based on knowledge grounded in research and passed on to new practitioners through educational programs sanctioned by the profession.

7. *Answer:* **D**

   Rationale: Commitment implies that professionals view their occupation as their life's work and part of their identity. Commitment is rewarded and honored.

8. Hospital billing practices lump charges for nursing care provided with hospital room charges.
   A. Autonomy.
   B. Vital service.
   C. Commitment.
   D. Specialized knowledge.

9. Direct and indirect supervision of nurses.
   A. Authority.
   B. Autonomy.
   C. Vital service.
   D. Commitment.

10. Physician approval is required for nursing procedures, standards of patient care, and nursing research.
    A. Authority.
    B. Autonomy.
    C. Commitment.
    D. Specialized knowledge.

Questions 11–13 are based on the following case. **Select the type of conflict management strategy used in each scenario.**
   A newly diagnosed adult chronic leukemia patient was hospitalized with a hemoglobin of 5.2 gm. After receiving 6 units of packed red blood cells over two days, the resident decides to discharge the patient. The discharge orders read: "Administer alpha-interferon 6 million units sq prior to discharge. Patient and family need to be taught how to administer at home."

11. The nurse argues that the patient is unfamiliar with his diagnosis, that the patient has not been observed for reactions to interferon, and that neither the patient nor his family know how to admix or administer the medication. The resident states, "That's not my problem, and, besides, I need that room for an emergency admission." The nurse fumes, walks away, and calls the leukemia attending physician.
    A. Competition.
    B. Avoidance.
    C. Accommodation.
    D. Compromise.

12. The nurse states that the patient is not prepared for discharge. The resident states that he cannot justify continuing the hospitalization of a patient with a hemoglobin of 9.2 gm and concludes, "That's not my problem." The nurse reiterates the reasons to postpone the discharge and states, "We can have the patient ready for discharge within twenty-four hours."
    A. Competition.
    B. Avoidance.
    C. Compromise.
    D. Collaboration.

13. The nurse tells herself, "That resident is a real jerk! His orders are ridiculous." The nurse administers the interferon and tells the oncoming nurse, "The patient needs interferon teaching."
    A. Avoidance.
    B. Accommodation.
    C. Compromise.
    D. Collaboration.

14. Benefits of collaborative relationships include which of the following?
    A. Concentrates power.
    B. Maximizes the unique skills of each person.
    C. Provides a single source of direction.
    D. Eliminates delegating to others.

15. In which of the following areas does nursing clearly differ from all other health disciplines?
    A. Holistic care of client.
    B. Practice-based expertise in behavioral and physical sciences.
    C. Lack of uniform preparation.
    D. Recognition of actual and potential problems.

16. Barriers to collaborative relationships include all of the following **EXCEPT**
    A. perceived threat to autonomy.
    B. identification with one's own profession.
    C. lack of administrative support.
    D. role confusion.

8. *Answer:* **B**

Rationale: A profession provides a highly valued service (vital service) that is of critical importance to society. In American society, a service of high value has a high price.

9. *Answer:* **B**

Rationale: Autonomous means self-regulating or self-governing.

10. *Answer:* **A**

Rationale: Authority is the power to act and implies that the action is independent.

11. *Answer:* **A**

Rationale: Competition = assertive + uncooperative.

12. *Answer:* **D**

Rationale: Collaboration = assertive + cooperative.

13. *Answer:* **A**

Rationale: Avoidance = unassertive + uncooperative.

14. *Answer:* **B**

Rationale: Collaborative relationships are characterized by shared power which is valued by all members. Slave–master relationships are characterized by one person giving commands that another will follow.

15. *Answer:* **C**

Rationale: Lack of uniform preparation of nurses creates role confusion.

16. *Answer:* **B**

Rationale: Identification with one's own profession is not considered a barrier to collaborative relationships, rather the impetus.

17. Which one of the following is **NOT** a characteristic of collaboration?
   A. Partnership.
   B. Commonality of goals.
   C. Shared power.
   D. Disparity of talents and efforts.

18. As a member of the interdisciplinary team, rather than an independent practitioner, the nurse must acknowledge and deal with which one of the following issues?
   A. Patient autonomy.
   B. Conflict between disciplines.
   C. Issues of territoriality and boundaries.
   D. Developing a dominant power base.

19. Select the **INCORRECT** statement.
   A. Society gives professional bodies the privilege to govern their own practice. In return, professions are accountable for managing their own functions.
   B. Self-regulation in assuring quality in performance and products is a hallmark of a profession.
   C. Peer review is a process by which society appraises the quality of care in accordance with established standards of practice.
   D. The peer review process includes both the appraisal of nursing care delivered by a group of nurses and the appraisal of an individual nurse.

There are three categories of standards: structure standards, process standards, and outcome standards. **Choose the type of standard that each of the following statements defines:**

20. Describes actions and behaviors for the provision of care, such as job descriptions, performance standards, procedures, protocols, and implementation strategies for nursing care plans.
   A. Structure standard.
   B. Process standard.
   C. Outcome standard.

21. Describes expected end results of nursing care, such as measurable changes in physiologic status, functional status, knowledge, and symptom control.
   A. Structure standard.
   B. Process standard.
   C. Outcome standard.

22. Describes conditions established to facilitate care, such as agency philosophy, nurse–patient ratio, qualifications of staff, equipment, and environment.
   A. Structure standard.
   B. Process standard.
   C. Outcome standard.

23. The following statements refer to potential occupational health standards. Select the **INCORRECT** statement.
   A. Heightened awareness and concern regarding the transmission of human immunodeficiency virus (HIV) served as an impetus for the implementation of "universal precautions."
   B. The Occupational Safety and Health Administration (OSHA) recommends that employers provide hepatitis B vaccines to at-risk employees.
   C. The occupational risk of contracting HIV is greater than the risk of contracting hepatitis B virus (HBV).
   D. OSHA states that a general duty of an employer is to furnish his employees with a place of employment free from recognized hazards causing or likely to cause death or serious illness.

24. Several governmental agencies have recommended that employers provide hepatitis B virus (HBV) vaccines to at-risk employees. Select the **INCORRECT** statement.
   A. Heptavax B® is recommended for persons allergic to yeast.
   B. The gluteus maximus is the recommended injection site for the administration of HBV vaccines.
   C. Post-exposure HBV vaccination is recommended.
   D. A series of HBV vaccine inoculations is more effective than a single vaccination.

17. *Answer:* **D**

Rationale: Collaboration is a true partnership in which the power on both sides is valued by both, with recognition and acceptance of separate and combined spheres of activity and responsibility and mutual safeguarding of the legitimate interests of both parties. Individuals in a true partnership believe that collaboration provides synergism of talents and efforts.

18. *Answer:* **C**

Rationale: As members of an interdisciplinary team, nurses must have a clear understanding of their roles and the roles of other disciplines in order to minimize distorted role expectations and avoid conflicts stemming from unequal distribution of power and influence.

19. *Answer:* **C**

Rationale: Peer review is a process by which professional nurses appraise the quality of care in accordance with established standards of practice.

20. *Answer:* **B**

Rationale: The defining statements for each standard are based upon literature and ANA/ONS standards.

21. *Answer:* **C**

Rationale: The defining statements for each standard are based upon literature and ANA/ONS standards.

22. *Answer:* **A**

Rationale: The defining statements for each standard are based upon literature and ANA/ONS standards.

23. *Answer:* **C**

Rationale: The occupational risk of contracting HBV is greater than the risk of contracting HIV.

24. *Answer:* **B**

Rationale: The deltoid muscle is the recommended injection site.

25. Select the **INCORRECT** statement.
   A. Acquired immunodeficiency syndrome (AIDS) is caused by the human immunodeficiency virus (HIV).
   B. HIV is transmitted via parenteral and mucous membrane exposure to infected blood or body fluid.
   C. The primary route of HIV occupational exposure of health care workers is via needle sticks.
   D. Health care workers infected with HIV should be excluded from caring for immunosuppressed patients.

26. Universal precaution guidelines advise that precautions be taken when the possibility of exposure to blood or body fluid exists. Select the **INCORRECT** statement.
   A. The type of anticipated exposure prescribes the type of protective barriers worn.
   B. Pregnant health care workers are not at higher risk to contract hepatitis B virus than are nonpregnant health care workers.
   C. Health care workers with exudative lesions or weeping dermatitis should double glove if direct patient care contact is anticipated.
   D. All patients should be assumed to be infectious for HIV and other blood-borne pathogens.

27. According to the *ANA/ONS Standards of Oncology Nursing Practice*, the role of the oncology nurse generalist in research includes all of the following activities **EXCEPT**
   A. conducting independent research.
   B. identifying research problems.
   C. evaluating research findings.
   D. incorporating applicable research into practice.

28. Which one of the following characteristics demonstrates an employment environment supportive of the nurse as the nurse improves the practice of oncology nursing through the review and application of research?
   A. Employing agency values nursing research.
   B. Employing agency supports nursing research by providing time, money resources, and recognition.
   C. Employing agency views the nurse generalist as a key person in identifying research problems.
   D. All of the above.

25. *Answer:* **D**

Rationale: Currently there are no exclusions of health care workers infected with HIV.

26. *Answer:* **C**

Rationale: Health care workers with exudative lesions or weeping dermatitis should refrain from direct patient care contact or handling soiled equipment until skin condition resolves. Pregnant health care workers are at no higher risk, and all health care workers should strictly adhere to protective practices.

27. *Answer:* **A**

Rationale: Conducting independent research is not a professional standard criterion established for the nurse generalist in oncology.

28. *Answer:* **D**

Rationale: All of the characteristics listed demonstrate support of nurse involvement with research and nursing research.

REFERENCES

American Nurses' Association, (1980). *Nursing: A Social Policy Statement*. Kansas City: American Nurses' Association.

American Nurses' Association and Oncology Nursing Society, (1987). *Standards of Oncology Nursing Practice*. Kansas City: American Nurses' Association.

Baggs J, Schmitt M, (1988). Collaboration Between Nurses and Physicians. *Image*. 20 (3): 145–149.

Center for Disease Control, (1987). Recommendations for Prevention of HIV Transmission in Health Care Settings. *MMWR*. 36 (2-S): 3S–17S.

Center for Disease Control, (1989). Guidelines for Prevention of Transmission of Human Immunodeficiency Virus and Hepatitis B Virus to Health Care and Public Safety Workers. *MMWR*. 38 (S-6): 1–39.

Center for Disease Control, (1990). Protection Against Viral Hepatitis. Recommendations of the Immunization Practices Advisory Committee. *MMWR* 39 (RR-2): 1–26.

Challela M, (1979). The Interdisciplinary Team: A Role Definition for Nursing. *Image*. 11 (1): 9–16.

Chenevert M, (1985). *ProNurse Handbook*. St. Louis: CV Mosby.

Cox A, (1981). The Development of Support Systems on Oncology Units. *Oncology Nursing Forum*. 8 (3): 31–35.

Cunningham M, (1992). Professional Issues in Cancer Care, in, Clark JC, McGee RF, (eds). *Core Curriculum for Oncology Nursing*, (2nd ed). Philadelphia: WB Saunders.

Department of Labor, (1987). Joint Advisory Notice; Department of Labor/Department of Health and Human Services; HBV/HIV. *Federal Register*. 52 (210): 41818–41823.

Gunning C, (1983). The Profession Itself as a Source of Stress, in, Jacobson S, McGrath H, (eds). *Nurses Under Stress*. New York: John Wiley and Sons.

Haber J, et al., (1982). *Comprehensive Psychiatric Nursing*. New York: McGraw-Hill.

Hall S, Wray L, (1989). Codependency. Nurses Who Give Too Much. *American Journal of Nursing*. 89 (11): 1456–1460.

Kilman R, Thomas K, (1977). Developing a Forced-choice Measure of Conflict-handling Behavior: The MODE Instrument. *Educational and Psychological Measurement*. 37 (4): 309–325.

Lazarus R, (1966). *Psychological Stress and the Coping Process*. New York: McGraw-Hill.

Marker C, (1987). The Marker Model: A Hierarchy for Nursing Standards. *Journal of Nursing Quality Assurance*. 1 (2): 7–20.

Patrick P, (1981). Burnout: Antecedents, Manifestations and Self-Care Strategies for Nurses, in, Marino L, (ed). *Cancer Nursing*. St. Louis: CV Mosby, pp. 113–138.

Prescott P, Brown S, (1985). Physician-nurse Relationships. *Annals of Internal Medicine*. 103 (1): 127–133.

Vachon M, et al., (1981). Measurement and Management of Stress in Health Professionals Working with Advanced Cancer Patients. *Death Education*. 1 (4): 365–375.

Webster JS, (1992). Sociodemographic and Attitudinal Changes Affecting Cancer Care, in, Clark JC, McGee RF, (eds). *Core Curriculum for Oncology Nursing*, (2nd ed). Philadelphia: WB Saunders.

8
Cancer Through the Life Span

Anne E. Belcher

Select the BEST answer for all of the following questions:

1. In response to a diagnosis of ineffective individual coping, the nurse might choose all of the following interventions **EXCEPT**
   A. evaluation, with the client, of the effectiveness of current coping strategies.
   B. instruction in relaxation, imagery, and other holistic stress reduction techniques.
   C. strengthening the client's social support system.
   D. providing referrals as needed to psychologist, social worker, etc.

2. Factors that affect the family's ability to cope with a diagnosis of cancer include all of the following **EXCEPT**
   A. developmental stage of members, e.g., empty nest.
   B. proximity of in-laws.
   C. members' responsibilities.
   D. preexisting stresses.

3. Mr. C told the nurse that "Everybody but me seems to be running my life since I got sick." Which of the following responses would be most appropriate in eliciting more information from Mr. C?
   A. "Why do you feel so powerless?"
   B. "What do you mean by that?"
   C. "Can you tell me about who is running your life?"
   D. "Tell me more about how that makes you feel."

4. Mr. J has recently been diagnosed with lung cancer. He stated, "I don't feel like I have any control over what is happening to me." Which of the following is an appropriate statement for the nurse to make?
   A. "Ask your doctor about your care and he will answer your questions."
   B. "We will develop a routine schedule for your care so you will know what to expect."
   C. "Ask your wife to let you do more things for yourself."
   D. "Let's spend some time talking about your feelings."

5. The person with an alteration in role performance would benefit from all the following nursing interventions **EXCEPT**
   A. assistance in setting priorities.
   B. identification of needed resources.
   C. avoidance of frustrating tasks.
   D. involvement of family as appropriate.

6. The nursing diagnosis that one would derive from an assessment of a person's difficulty in meeting developmental tasks is
   A. diversional activity, deficit.
   B. growth and development, altered.
   C. role performance, altered.
   D. knowledge deficit.

1. *Answer:* **C**

    Rationale: While the nurse may help the client to identify the current social support system, only the client can determine the need to, and/or the ways in which to, strengthen it.

2. *Answer:* **B**

    Rationale: While the nearness of in-laws may be viewed as affecting family functioning, in the presence of a cancer diagnosis, it would more correctly be viewed as a preexisting stressor.

3. *Answer:* **D**

    Rationale: Use an open-ended question to elicit individual perceptions of the response without jumping to conclusions of a diagnosis of powerlessness.

4. *Answer:* **D**

    Rationale: To plan care, the nurse would need to have additional information regarding the specific areas of perceived loss of control.

5. *Answer:* **C**

    Rationale: Avoidance of frustrating tasks may only increase the patient's sense of inadequacy and/or helplessness.

6. *Answer:* **C**

    Rationale: Inability to meet one's developmental tasks has a direct impact on one's role performance in many ways, such as worker, spouse, and parent.

7. The priority data to collect when assessing a person's developmental level are
   A. completed developmental tasks.
   B. tasks of an ongoing nature.
   C. perceived impact of cancer on developmental goals.
   D. goals identified for attainment in the future.

8. At which developmental level is the individual adjusting to the greatest number of losses?
   A. Adolescence.
   B. Early adulthood.
   C. Middle adulthood.
   D. Older adulthood.

9. Which of the following is **NOT** a developmental task of older adulthood (over 55 years of age)?
   A. Adjusting to retirement.
   B. Assisting adolescent children.
   C. Adjusting to death of a spouse.
   D. Adapting social roles in a flexible way.

10. Which of the following is **NOT** a developmental task of middle adulthood (30–55 years)?
   A. Taking on civic responsibility.
   B. Adjusting to aging parents.
   C. Relating to one's spouse as a person.
   D. Adjusting to physiologic changes.

11. Which of the following is **NOT** a developmental task of early adulthood (18–30 years)?
   A. Selecting a mate.
   B. Starting a family.

   C. Developing leisure activities.
   D. Initiating an occupation.

12. Which of the following is **NOT** a characteristic of family relationships?
   A. Cohesion.
   B. Expressiveness.
   C. Conflict.
   D. Diagnosis.

13. Factors to consider when assessing a person's living conditions include all of the following **EXCEPT**
   A. type of housing.
   B. ownership versus rental.
   C. number of occupants.
   D. level of employment.

14. Poverty causes all of the following barriers to cancer prevention, early detection, and diagnosis **EXCEPT**
   A. substandard housing.
   B. chronic malnutrition.
   C. ethnic superstition.
   D. inadequate education.

15. The myth held by the general public that has the most adverse effect on its awareness of cancer in the elderly is which of the following?
   A. Elderly persons are senile or demented.
   B. Older persons are generally unhealthy.
   C. The aged are unable to care for themselves.
   D. Aging results in inevitable deterioration.

7. *Answer:* **A**

Rationale: Assessment focuses on developmental level, not the patient's goals.

8. *Answer:* **D**

Rationale: Older adulthood includes decreasing physical strength, retirement, death of spouse, and death of friends.

9. *Answer:* **B**

Rationale: Assisting adolescent children is a task of middle adulthood.

10. *Answer:* **A**

Rationale: Taking on civic responsibility is a task of early adulthood.

11. *Answer:* **C**

Rationale: Developing leisure activities is defined as a middle adulthood task.

12. *Answer:* **D**

Rationale: To the extent that diagnosis is one aspect of the decision-making process, it can be considered an aspect of family functioning, but it does not define relationships to the extent that the other terms do.

13. *Answer:* **D**

Rationale: While level of employment may indicate the type or condition of housing, it is a less direct measure of living conditions than are the other criteria.

14. *Answer:* **C**

Rationale: There is no evidence that poverty per se generates ethnic superstition, although difficulty in accessing the health care system might cause the person to suspect prejudice as a factor.

15. *Answer:* **D**

Rationale: While many elderly persons are unhealthy, the perception that deterioration in health is unavoidable prevents the public from viewing change in health status as a possible indication of cancer.

REFERENCES

Belcher A, (1992). Factors Affecting Responses to the Risk for or Actual Diagnosis of Cancer, in, Clark JC, McGee RF, (eds). *Core Curriculum for Oncology Nursing,* (2nd ed). Philadelphia: WB Saunders.

Dugan SO, Scallion LM, (1984). The Older Adult, in, McIntire SN, Cioppa AL, (eds). *Cancer Nursing: A Developmental Approach.* New York: John Wiley and Sons, pp. 225–253.

Germino B, (1991). Cancer amd the Family, in, Baird SB, McCorkle R, Grant M, (eds). *Cancer Nursing: A Comprehensive Textbook.* Philadephia: WB Saunders, pp. 38–44.

Lewis FM, (1986). The Impact of Cancer on the Family: A Critical Analysis of the Research Literature. *Patient Education and Counseling.* 8 (3): 269–289.

Kim MJ, McFarland GK, McLane AM, (1987). *Pocket Guide to Nursing Diagnoses,* (2nd ed). St. Louis: CV Mosby.

McIntire SN, (1991). Developmental Process, in, Baird SB, McCorkle R, Grant M, (eds). *Cancer Nursing: A Comprehensive Textbook.* Philadephia: WB Saunders, pp. 55–60.

McIntire SN, (1984). The Adult, in, McIntire SN, Cioppa AL, (eds). *Cancer Nursing: A Developmental Approach.* New York: John Wiley and Sons, pp. 206–223.

Thorne SE, (1988). Helpful and Unhelpful Communications in Cancer Care: The Patient Perspective. *Oncology Nursing Forum.* 15 (2): 167–172.

Webster JS, (1992). Sociodemographic and Attitudinal Changes Affecting Cancer Care, in, Clark JC, McGee RF, (eds). *Core Curriculum for Oncology Nursing,* (2nd ed). Philadelphia: WB Saunders.

9
Pathophysiology of Cancer

General Concepts
Deborah L. Volker

The Process of Carcinogenesis
Deborah L. Volker

General Concepts
Deborah L. Volker

Select the BEST answer for all of the following questions:

1. Aneuploidy means that many malignant cells have an abnormal amount of
   A. DNA.
   B. chromosomes.
   C. nuclei.
   D. mitochondria.

2. Chronic irritation from cigarette smoke can cause bronchial epithelium to change from ciliated pseudostratified columnar epithelium to stratified squamous epithelium. This change is termed
   A. hyperplasia.
   B. metaplasia.
   C. dysplasia.
   D. anaplasia.

3. Failure of systemic therapy for cancer is best explained by the tumor property of
   A. heterogeneity.
   B. anaplasia.
   C. necrosis.
   D. metastasis.

4. The loss of contact inhibition allows a malignant cell to
   A. invade adjacent tissue.
   B. transform into progressively primitive forms.
   C. adhere to other malignant cells.
   D. resist many forms of treatment.

1. *Answer:* **B**

   Rationale: An abnormal number of chromosomes, termed *aneuploidy,* is a typical change present in the nuclei of cancer cells.

2. *Answer:* **B**

   Rationale: Metaplasia refers to the replacement of one mature cell type by another.

3. *Answer:* **A**

   Rationale: Although all of the options describe properties of malignant tumors, the problem of heterogeneity best answers the question because it refers to the marked variations between individual cells within a tumor. These variations cause the tumor to have varying susceptibilities to treatment.

4. *Answer:* **A**

   Rationale: Unchecked migratory activity due to a loss of contact inhibition allows malignant cells to spread locally by invading adjacent tissue.

5. Use of alternating, multiple-drug chemotherapeutic regimens is designed to overcome tumor
   A. homogeneity.
   B. heterogeneity.
   C. differentiation.
   D. initiation.

6. Your patient had a biopsy of a mass in his leg. The pathology report confirms that it is a lipoma. You anticipate that he will require
   A. local excision and a diagnostic work-up for metastases.
   B. local excision and radiation therapy.
   C. local excision and chemotherapy.
   D. none of the above.

7. Multiple myeloma is a malignancy that arises from
   A. T-lymphocytes.
   B. plasma cells.
   C. myelocytes.
   D. monocytes.

8. A malignant tumor that originates in connective tissue is a
   A. papilloma.
   B. fibroma.
   C. carcinoma.
   D. sarcoma.

9. The type of tissue from which bronchogenic carcinoma arises is
   A. epithelial.
   B. connective.
   C. muscle.
   D. endothelial.

10. An adenocarcinoma arises from
    A. squamous cells.
    B. glandular epithelium.
    C. connective tissue.
    D. endothelial tissue.

11. Which of the following is a benign neoplasm of epithelial origin?
    A. Carcinoma.
    B. Fibroma.
    C. Sarcoma.
    D. Adenoma.

12. Sarcomas arise from
    A. mesenchymal tissue.
    B. lymphoid cells.
    C. squamous cells.
    D. epithelial tissue.

13. A rhabdomyosarcoma arises from
    A. smooth muscle.
    B. skeletal muscle.
    C. collagen fibers.
    D. fibrocartilage.

5. *Answer:* **B**

Rationale: Because numerous heterogeneous subpopulations of cells tend to exist within a single tumor, and because these subpopulations have differing susceptibilities to different drugs, a multi-drug approach is more effective than a single drug. Alternating regimens may be more successful in that they decrease the chance that resistant genetic alterations will arise after repetitive exposure to the same drug regimen.

6. *Answer:* **D**

Rationale: A lipoma is a benign tumor of fatty origin. Thus, it will not become invasive or metastatic.

7. *Answer:* **B**

Rationale: Multiple myeloma is a hematologic malignancy that arises in plasma cells.

8. *Answer:* **D**

Rationale: Malignant tumors of mesenchymal origin are sarcomas. Connective tissue, such as bone, fat, and cartilage, are all of mesenchymal origin.

9. *Answer:* **A**

Rationale: The term carcinoma is used to describe malignancies of epithelial origin.

10. *Answer:* **B**

Rationale: Malignancies that arise from glandular epithelium are termed adenocarcinomas.

11. *Answer:* **D**

Rationale: Benign tumors typically end with the suffix "oma"; tumors that arise from glandular epithelium begin with the prefix "adeno".

12. *Answer:* **A**

Rationale: The root "sarc" refers to a malignancy of mesenchymal origin.

13. *Answer:* **B**

Rationale: The term "rhabdo" refers to striated or skeletal muscle.

REFERENCES

Cook MB, (1990). Multiple Myeloma, in, Groenwald SL, Frogge MH, Goodman M, Yarbro CH, (eds). *Cancer Nursing Principles and Practice*, (2nd ed). Boston: Jones and Bartlett, pp. 990–998.

Cotran RS, Kumar V, Robbins SL, (1989). *Robbins Pathologic Basis of Disease*, (4th ed). Philadelphia: WB Saunders.

Gallucci BB, (1991). Cancer Biology: Molecular and Cellular Aspects, in, Baird SB, McCorkle R, Grant M, (eds). *Cancer Nursing: A Comprehensive Textbook*. Philadephia: WB Saunders, pp. 115–129.

Heppner GH, Miller BE, (1989). Therapeutic Implications of Tumor Heterogeneity. *Seminars in Oncology*. 16: 91–105.

Hubbard SM, Liotta LA, (1991). The Biology of Metastases, in, Baird SB, McCorkle R, Grant M, (eds). *Cancer Nursing: A Comprehensive Textbook*. Philadephia: WB Saunders, pp. 130–142.

Kupchella CE, (1990). Cellular Biology of Cancer, in, Groenwald SL, Frogge MH, Goodman M, Yarbro CH, (eds). *Cancer Nursing Principles and Practice*, (2nd ed). Boston: Jones and Bartlett, pp. 43–57.

Lieberman MW, Lebovitz RM, (1990). Neoplasia, in, Kissane JM, (ed). *Anderson's Pathology*, (9th ed). New York: Plenum Press, pp. 566–614.

O'Mary SS, (1990). Diagnostic Evaluation, Classification, and Staging, in, Groenwald SL, Frogge MH, Goodman M, Yarbro CH, (eds). *Cancer Nursing Principles and Practice*, (2nd ed). Boston: Jones and Bartlett, pp. 161–174.

Salmon SE, Cassady JR, (1989). Plasma Cell Neoplasms, in, DeVita VT, Hellman S, Rosenberg S, (eds). *Cancer Principles and Practice of Oncology*, (3rd ed). Philadelphia: JB Lippincott, pp. 1853–1895.

Schnipper LE, (1986). Clinical Applications of Tumor-cell Heterogeneity. *New England Journal of Medicine*. 314: 1423–1431.

Sirica AE, (1989). Classification of Neoplasms, in, Sirica AE, (ed). *The Pathology of Neoplasia*. New York: Plenum Press, pp. 25–38.

Strohl RA, (1992). Implications of Diagnosis and Staging in Treatment Goals and Strategies, in, Clark JC, McGee RF, (eds). *Core Curriculum for Oncology Nursing*, (2nd ed). Philadelphia: WB Saunders.

Volker DL, (1992). Pathophysiology of Cancer, in, Clark JC, McGee RF, (eds). *Core Curriculum for Oncology Nursing*, (2nd ed). Philadelphia: WB Saunders.

Woodruff M, (1990). *Cellular Variation and Adaptation in Cancer*. New York: Oxford University Press.

The Process of Carcinogenesis

Deborah Volker

Select the BEST answer for all of the following questions:

1. In the process of carcinogenesis, a proto-oncogene may be activated, leading to
    A. uncontrolled cell proliferation.
    B. suppressed cell growth.
    C. defective anti-oncogene formation.
    D. uncontrolled anti-oncogene formation.

2. Mrs. J has a history of receiving cyclophosphamide and radiation therapy for Hodgkin's disease. She is now at risk for developing
    A. melanoma.
    B. colon cancer.
    C. leukemia.
    D. osteosarcoma.

3. The use of condoms and spermicides during sexual intercourse may decrease the transmission of which initiating factor for cervical cancer?
    A. Epstein-Barr virus.
    B. Cytomegalovirus.
    C. Human papilloma virus (HPV).
    D. Human immunodeficiency virus.

4. Carcinogenesis refers to the process of _____ _____ of normal cells to malignant cells.
    A. migration
    B. degradation
    C. differentiation
    D. transformation

5. Green and yellow vegetables contain retinols that can reverse cell
    A. transformation.
    B. metastasis.
    C. inhibition.
    D. synthesis.

6. According to the immune surveillance theory, tumor cells may escape destruction by
    A. overwhelming the immune system with a large tumor cell burden.
    B. expressing cell surface antigens that resemble normal or "self" antigens.
    C. expressing nonimmunogenic antigens.
    D. all of the above.

7. The immune system may be able to recognize and destroy cancer cells due to the presence of
    A. endotoxins.
    B. embryonic oncogenes.
    C. tumor-associated antigens.
    D. anaplastic antibodies.

8. Currently, tumor-associated antigens, such as alpha-fetoprotein and carcinoembryonic antigen, are used to
    A. pinpoint a tumor's location.
    B. screen for tumors in the general population.
    C. monitor a patient's response to treatment.
    D. all of the above.

9. A tumor mass increases in size because
    A. the rate of cell death continually declines throughout the life of the tumor.
    B. the rate of cell production is greater than the rate of cell death.
    C. the rate of cell proliferation is more rapid than in normal tissue.
    D. all of the above.

10. The smallest clinically detectable tumor mass is approximately
    A. 0.01 cm.
    B. 0.10 cm.
    C. 1.00 cm.
    D. 10.0 cm.

1. *Answer:* **A**

   Rationale: Activation of a proto-oncogene is believed to be a key step in tumor growth. Proto-oncogenes serve as important regulators of orderly cell proliferation.

2. *Answer:* **C**

   Rationale: Both radiation therapy and alkylating chemotherapeutic agents are known carcinogens that can cause leukemia. Leukemia has long been recognized as a therapy-related malignancy.

3. *Answer:* **C**

   Rationale: Although use of condoms can decrease the transmission of all of the viruses listed, and all of the viruses are known to be viral carcinogens, HPV is the only virus listed known to be associated with cervical cancer.

4. *Answer:* **D**

   Rationale: Cells undergo a number of transformations as they become malignant.

5. *Answer:* **A**

   Rationale: Dietary retinols have been shown to be able to reverse the process of chemical carcinogenesis. The process of carcinogenesis is characterized by neoplastic transformation of the cell.

6. *Answer:* **D**

   Rationale: The immune surveillance mechanism is thought to provide some protection against the proliferation of malignant cells. This system can fail, however, due to numerous factors, including all of those listed above.

7. *Answer:* **C**

   Rationale: The underlying concept of tumor immunology is that the immune system can recognize foreign, or "non-self" surface antigens on cancer cells.

8. *Answer:* **C**

   Rationale: When used as tumor markers, tumor-associated antigens are not specific enough to pinpoint tumor location, nor are they specific enough to be used as a screening tool for the general population. They *can* be used to assess disease response.

9. *Answer:* **B**

   Rationale: Tumors grow because the rate of cell production is greater than the rate of cell death.

10. *Answer:* **C**

    Rationale: By the time a tumor mass is clinically detectable (by physical or radiologic exam), it will have reached a size of about 1.00 cm (or 1 gm in weight).

11. Tamoxifen citrate may be used to treat a hormonally dependent breast cancer, based on the principle that
   A. enhancing hormone availability to normal cells will decrease availability to cancer cells.
   B. suppressing hormone availability to cancer cells will increase their susceptibility to chemotherapy.
   C. suppressing hormone availability to cancer cells can suppress their growth.
   D. enhancing hormone availability to cancer cells will suppress DNA synthesis and result in cell death.

12. Cancers that are most vulnerable to chemotherapy tend to have a relatively high
   A. degree of heterogeneity.
   B. tumor burden.
   C. growth fraction.
   D. level of fibronectin.

13. A pathology report notes the presence of hyperplasia. This means that the cells examined have an abnormal increase in
   A. number.
   B. invasiveness.
   C. size.
   D. differentiation.

14. "Carcinoma in situ" means that the cancer has not yet become
   A. malignant.
   B. transformed.
   C. invasive.
   D. metastatic.

15. A systemic approach to the treatment of cancer is often necessary because
   A. local invasion is best controlled this way.
   B. tumor growth will continue exponentially after diagnosis.
   C. tumor cells will increase their doubling time.
   D. metastatic spread has likely occurred before diagnosis.

16. Metastatic spread of malignant cells most often occurs in all the following sites **EXCEPT**
   A. the lung.
   B. the liver.
   C. the kidney.
   D. the bone.

17. Specific tumors tend to metastasize to specific target organs because
   A. the immune system selectively destroys metastatic deposits to nontarget organs.
   B. therapeutic levels of chemotherapy may not be achieved in target organs.
   C. target organs are more vascular, thus providing more nutrients to metastatic cells.
   D. metastatic cells may be able to elicit necessary growth factors only in target organs.

11. *Answer:* **C**

Rationale: Many breast cancers require estrogen for growth. Reduction in hormone levels via an antiestrogen compound (tamoxifen) can suppress or reduce tumor growth.

12. *Answer:* **C**

Rationale: Most chemotherapeutic agents exert their greatest effect on cycling cells. Thus, cancers with a high growth fraction, or relatively high proportion of cells in the proliferative pool, are most vulnerable to the effects of chemotherapy.

13. *Answer:* **A**

Rationale: The term "hyperplasia" refers to an increase in the number of cells.

14. *Answer:* **C**

Rationale: "Carcinoma in situ" is a cancer that possesses the cytologic features of malignant, transformed cells but has not yet invaded the basement membrane.

15. *Answer:* **D**

Rationale: Because metastatic spread has likely occurred prior to diagnosis, a local approach to therapy will not treat cancer cells at distant sites.

16. *Answer:* **C**

Rationale: Tumors tend to metastasize to particular, predictable sites. The most common sites include lymph nodes, bone, lung, liver, and the brain.

17. *Answer:* **D**

Rationale: Although many hypotheses exist to explain the organ specificity of metastasis, response D is the only choice of the four that is currently supported by experimental studies.

REFERENCES

Alkire K, Groenwald SL, (1990). Relation of the Immune System to Cancer, in, Groenwald SL, Frogge MH, Goodman M, Yarbro CH, (eds). *Cancer Nursing Principles and Practice*, (2nd ed). Boston: Jones and Bartlett, pp. 72–88.

Cotran RS, Kumar V, Robbins SL, (1989). *Robbins Pathologic Basis of Disease*, (4th ed). Philadelphia: WB Saunders.

Collins P, (1990). Tumor Markers and Screening Tools in Cancer Detection. *Nursing Clinics of North America*. 25: 283–290.

Dawson M, Moore M, (1989). Tumor Immunology, in, Roitt M, Brostoff J, Male DK, (eds). *Immunology*, (2nd ed). St. Louis: CV Mosby.

Fidler IJ, Nicolson GL, (1987). The Process of Cancer Invasion and Metastasis. *Cancer Bulletin*. 39: 126–131.

Gallucci B, (1987). The Immune System and Cancer. *Oncology Nursing Forum*. 14 (6): 3–12.

Goodman M, (1988). Concepts of Hormonal Manipulation in the Treatment of Cancer. *Oncology Nursing Forum*. 15: 639–647.

Greenwald P, (1989). Principles of Cancer Prevention: Diet and Nutrition, in, DeVita VT, Hellman S, Rosenberg S, (eds). *Cancer Principles and Practice of Oncology*, (3rd ed). Philadelphia: JB Lippincott, pp. 167–180.

Hubbard SM, Liotta LA, (1991). The Biology of Metastases, in, Baird SB, McCorkle R, Grant M, (eds). *Cancer Nursing: A Comprehensive Textbook*. Philadephia: WB Saunders, pp. 130–146.

Killion JJ, Fidler IJ, (1989). The Biology of Tumor Metastasis. *Seminars in Oncology*. 16: 106–115.

Lilley L, Schaffer S, (1990). Human Papillomavirus: A Sexually Transmitted Disease With Carcinogenic Potential. *Cancer Nursing*. 13: 366–372.

Liotta LA, Strack ML, Wewer UM, Schiffman E, (1989). Tumor Invasion and Metastases: Biochemical Mechanisms, in, Sirica AE, (ed). *The Pathobiology of Neoplasia*. New York: Plenum Press, pp. 533–546.

Litherland S, Jackson I, (1988). Antioestrogens in the Management of Hormone Dependent Breast Cancer. *Cancer Treatment Reports*. 15: 183–194.

Mettlin C, Mirand AL, (1991). The Causes of Cancer, in, Baird SB, McCorkle R, Grant M, (eds). *Cancer Nursing: A Comprehensive Textbook*. Philadephia: WB Saunders, pp. 104–114.

Nicolson G, (1988). Organ Specificity of Tumor Metastases: Role of Preferential Adhesion, Invasion, and Growth of Malignant Cells at Specific Secondary Sites. *Cancer Metastasis Review*. 7: 143–188.

Pape LH, (1988). Therapy-related Acute Leukemia: An Overview. *Cancer Nursing*. 11: 295–302.

Sell S, (1987). *Immunology, Immunopathology, and Immunity*, (4th ed). New York: Elsevier.

Tannock IF, (1989). Principles of Cell Proliferation: Cell Kinetics, in, DeVita VT, Hellman S, Rosenberg S, (eds). *Cancer Principles and Practice of Oncology*, (3rd ed). Philadelphia: WB Saunders, pp. 3–13.

Tucker MA, Coleman CN, Cox RS, Varghese A, Rosenberg S, (1988). Risk of Second Cancers after Treatment for Hodgkin's Disease. *New England Journal of Medicine*. 318: 76–81.

Vaughn TL, McTiernan A, (1986). Diet in the Etiology of Cancer. *Seminars in Oncology Nursing*. 2 (1): 3–13.

Virji M, Mercer D, Herberman R, (1988). Tumor Markers in Cancer Diagnosis and Prognosis. *CA*. 38 (3): 104–126.

Volker DL, (1992). Pathophysiology of Cancer, in, Clark JC, McGee RF, (eds). *Core Curriculum for Oncology Nursing*, (2nd ed). Philadelphia: WB Saunders.

Woodruff M, (1990). *Cellular Variation and Adaptation in Cancer: Biologic Basis and Therapeutic Consequences*. New York: Oxford University Press.

Yarbro JW, (1990). Carcinogenesis, in, Groenwald SL, Frogge MH, Goodman M, Yarbro CH, (eds). *Cancer Nursing Principles and Practice*, (2nd ed). Boston: Jones and Bartlett, pp. 31–42.

10
Cancer Epidemiology

Karen Smith Blesch and Marilyn Frank-Stromborg

Select the BEST answer for all of the following questions:

1. Epidemiology is primarily concerned with disease as it occurs in
   A. epidemics.
   B. human populations.
   C. individual persons.
   D. families.

2. An epidemiologic study collects data about the occurrence of breast cancer around the world and discovers that breast cancer is more common in American women than in Japanese women. This kind of study would best be described as
   A. an analytic intervention study.
   B. an analytic observational study.
   C. a descriptive observational study.
   D. an observational intervention study.

3. An epidemiologic study of the occurrence of invasive cervical cancer finds that this cancer occurs more frequently in women of lower socioeconomic status than in women of higher socioeconomic status. This information is useful for
   A. generating hypotheses regarding causes of cervical cancer.
   B. testing hypotheses regarding causes of cervical cancer.
   C. identifying new treatments for cervical cancer.
   D. describing the natural history of cervical cancer.

4. The primary goal of cancer epidemiology is to
   A. identify which cancers can be cured and cure them.
   B. predict who will get cancer so that health services are available when they get sick.
   C. identify factors that cause cancer so that cancer can be prevented.
   D. get people to avoid exposure to known and suspected carcinogens.

5. Town X has an adult population of 5000. Over a period of one year there were 35 newly diagnosed cases of colon cancer in town X. These were added to 145 already-existing cases. The **INCIDENCE RATE** of colon cancer in town X is
   A. 145/5000 per year.
   B. 35/5000 per year.
   C. 35/4855 per year.
   D. 180/5000 per year.

6. Town X has an adult population of 5000. Over a period of one year there were 35 newly diagnosed cases of colon cancer in town X. These were added to 145 already-existing cases. The **PREVALENCE RATE** of colon cancer in town X at this point in time is
   A. 145/5000.
   B. 35/5000.
   C. 35/4855.
   D. 180/5000.

1. *Answer:* **B**

    Rationale: Epidemiology is a population-based science.

2. *Answer:* **C**

    Rationale: No intervention done—not an intervention study (A, D); no analysis done—not analytic (B); a strictly descriptive study, observation methodology.

3. *Answer:* **A**

    Rationale: This is a descriptive study and uses descriptive data. This is the first step toward the generation of a hypothesis.

4. *Answer:* **C**

    Rationale: This is the purpose of cancer epidemiology and allows discrimination among the primary goal of epidemiology, and other,

secondary goals. The secondary goals are best achieved by disciplines other than epidemiology.

5. *Answer:* **C**

    Rationale: This question tests one's ability to calculate incidence rate as defined and differentiate between incidence and prevalence:

$$\text{Incidence} = \frac{\text{Number of new cases of a specific disease in 1 year}}{\text{Population at risk in the same year}}$$

6. *Answer:* **D**

    Rationale: This question tests one's ability to calculate prevalence rate as defined and differentiate between incidence and prevalence:

$$\text{Prevalence} = \frac{\text{Number of cases (new + existing)}}{\text{Number of persons in the population}}$$

7. It is important to collect and analyze cancer prevalence statistics because
   - A. they give a clear picture of the risk of developing cancer.
   - B. they are useful for testing hypotheses regarding the etiology of cancer.
   - C. they provide information for allocation of health resources for persons with cancer.
   - D. they provide the best evidence for the effectiveness of certain cancer treatments.

8. Smoking restrictions in public areas are an example of primary prevention through intervention targeted at the
   - A. host.
   - B. agent.
   - C. environment.
   - D. agent and the environment.

9. By lowering their intake of dietary fat and increasing their intake of fiber, persons are hoping to prevent cancer by directly altering
   - A. their susceptibility to disease.
   - B. their exposure to presumed agents of disease.
   - C. the presumed agents of disease.
   - D. their susceptibility and exposure.

10. Many persons who smoke cigarettes never develop lung cancer. The **BEST** explanation for this phenomenon is
   - A. smokers develop other smoking-related diseases and die before they develop lung cancer.
   - B. there is an unknown factor that predisposes persons to becoming smokers and that also predisposes them to lung cancer.
   - C. there are complex interactions between cigarette smoke, the individual person, the environment, and lifestyle that determine whether or not lung cancer develops.
   - D. some smokers may prevent lung cancer by eating diets that contain large amounts of nutrients known to prevent lung cancer.

11. Low-tar and low-nicotine cigarettes presume to reduce lung cancer risk by
   - A. altering the agent.
   - B. altering the host.
   - C. altering the environment.
   - D. all of the above.

12. Among Americans, where does cancer (all sites) rank as a cause of death?
   - A. First.
   - B. Second.
   - C. Third.
   - D. Fourth.

13. Which of the following age/sex groups has the lowest cancer mortality?
   - A. Males aged 1–14.
   - B. Females aged 1–14.
   - C. Males aged 15–34.
   - D. Females aged 15–34.

14. Among American women aged 55–74, which cancer site is the leading cause of cancer mortality?
   - A. Breast.
   - B. Lung.
   - C. Colon and rectum.
   - D. Ovary.

15. Which of the following age/sex groups has the highest cancer mortality?
   - A. Females aged 35–74.
   - B. Males aged 35–74.
   - C. Males aged 75 and over.
   - D. Females aged 75 and over.

16. Which of the following is the primary force propelling cancer into the top four leading causes of death in the latter half of this century?
   - A. Changes in cancer treatment.
   - B. Reduced mortality from infectious disease.
   - C. Increasing air and water pollution.
   - D. Exposure to carcinogenic chemicals in the food supply.

17. The leading cause of death from cancer in both men and women over the age of 35 is
   - A. colorectal cancer.
   - B. lung cancer.
   - C. cancer of the urologic system.
   - D. leukemia.

7.   *Answer:* **C**

Rationale: Health resources can be better allocated when the total number of individuals affected is known and analyzed.

8.   *Answer:* **C**

Rationale: Removal of the agent (cigarette smoke) alters the environment of the host. There are no direct alterations in the host or of the agent.

9.   *Answer:* **B**

Rationale: While susceptibility may be indirectly affected by dietary changes, the direct effect is to remove the exposure.

10.   *Answer:* **C**

Rationale: C is the best response because it is the broadest, subsuming all the others. While the other three responses may be true to a certain extent (especially A), they do not provide a complete explanation. Response B is the old tobacco-industry argument and should be recognized as such.

11.   *Answer:* **A**

Rationale: The agent is cigarette smoke, which is directly altered. Any effects on the host or environment are indirect.

12.   *Answer:* **B**

Rationale: Heart disease is the leading cause of death; cancer is second.

13.   *Answer:* **C**

Rationale: Cancer is the fifth leading cause of mortality in males aged 15–34, behind accidents, suicide, homicide, and HIV infection, in that order.

14.   *Answer:* **B**

Rationale: Age distinction is important. Colorectal cancer is the leading cause of death in women aged 75 and over. In women aged 35–54, breast cancer is the leading cause of cancer mortality.

15.   *Answer:* **A**

Rationale: This is due to the impact of the occurrence of breast, lung, and GYN malignancies in this age group.

16.   *Answer:* **B**

Rationale: Reductions in one cause of death lead to increases in other causes of death.

17.   *Answer:* **B**

Rationale: Lung cancer is the leading cause of death in both sexes.

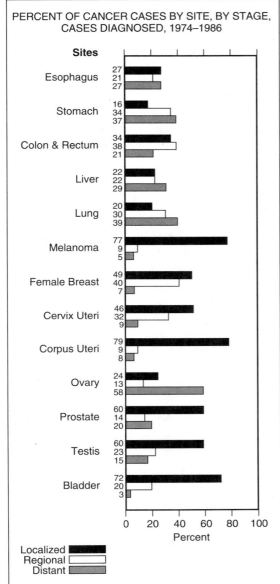

PERCENT OF CANCER CASES BY SITE, BY STAGE, CASES DIAGNOSED, 1974–1986

Localized ▉
Regional ☐
Distant ▨

Note: This chart is based on cases diagnosed in 1974–1986 and represents the latest data available on survival by stage. Staging is by the historical classification, which differs somewhat from the American Joint Committee on Cancer (AJCC) staging used in previous years.

Source: Cancer Statistics Branch, National Cancer Institute.

FIGURE 10–1. Percent of cancer cases by site, by stage, and cases diagnosed, 1974–1986. (Redrawn from Cancer Statistics Branch, National Cancer Institute, in, Boring CC, Squires TS, *Cancer Statistics, 1991. CA.* 41 (1): 21.

18. Refer to Figure 10–1. From 1974 to 1986, most cases of prostate cancer were diagnosed at which stage?
   A. Localized.
   B. Regional.
   C. Distant.
   D. Unknown.

19. Which of the following is **NOT** among the top five cancer sites affecting American women aged 15 years and over?
   A. Breast.
   B. Colon and rectum.
   C. Cervix.
   D. Lung.

20. Which of the following cancers **OCCURS** most frequently among adults in the United States?
   A. Breast cancer.
   B. Prostate cancer.
   C. Lung cancer.
   D. Colorectal cancer.

21. Choose the answer that correctly ranks, in order of their frequency of occurrence, the top three cancer sites in American males.
   A. Lung, prostate, colorectal.
   B. Lung, colorectal, prostate.
   C. Prostate, lung, colorectal.
   D. Colorectal, lung, prostate.

22. Of all the cancers that affect women, which has shown the largest increase in incidence in the past two decades?
   A. Colon cancer.
   B. Ovarian cancer.
   C. Breast cancer.
   D. Lung cancer.

23. Which one of the following cancer sites has experienced a dramatic decline in incidence in the past two decades?
   A. Prostate.
   B. Female breast.
   C. Stomach.
   D. Colon.

18. *Answer:* **A**

Rationale: This question tests one's ability to correctly read and interpret epidemiologic information presented in graph format.

19. *Answer:* **C**

Rationale: Cervical cancer accounts for less than 3% of cancers in women, compared to 32%, 14% and 11%, respectively, for the other cancers listed.

20. *Answer:* **A**

Rationale: In 1991, breast cancer incidence was estimated to be 32%; prostate cancer, 22%; lung cancer, 19% M, 11% F; and colorectal, 14%.

21. *Answer:* **C**

Rationale: Prostate cancer incidence = 22%, lung cancer = 19%, colorectal cancer = 14%, estimated in 1991.

22. *Answer:* **D**

Rationale: Lung cancer showed a 95% increase from 1973–1987, compared to a 23% increase for breast cancer. Ovarian cancer has declined, and colon cancer has increased only slightly.

23. *Answer:* **C**

Rationale: Cancer of the stomach incidence decreased from 9.5% in 1973 to 7.1% in 1986. An increased incidence was noted in the other three cancer sites listed.

24. In this century, which cancer site has shown the largest increase in incidence in both men and women?
  A. Lung and bronchus.
  B. Colorectal.
  C. Head and neck.
  D. Stomach.

25. From 1955–1970, the incidence of carcinoma in situ of the uterine cervix nearly quintupled. The most likely explanation for this trend is
  A. women developed cervical cancer at a faster rate than previously.
  B. widespread use of the Papanicolaou smear uncovered many previously undiagnosed cases.
  C. widespread use of oral contraceptives placed many women at risk for developing cervical cancer.
  D. the population of women at risk for developing cervical cancer increased.

26. Which site is *the leader* in cancer mortality for American adult females?
  A. Breast.
  B. Lung.
  C. Cervix.
  D. Ovary.

27. Select the best definition of "cancer survival rate" from those given below.
  A. The percent of persons who die of cancer over a given period of time.
  B. The percent of persons with cancer who live five years.
  C. The proportion of a defined group of patients with cancer who are still alive after a given period of time.
  D. The percent of persons with cancer who die within five years.

24.   *Answer:* **A**

Rationale: Both men and women have an increased incidence of lung cancer because of smoking habits.

25.   *Answer:* **B**

Rationale: The Pap smear is an effective early detection technique.

26.   *Answer:* **B**

Rationale: Lung cancer mortality surpassed breast cancer mortality in 1988.

27.   *Answer:* **C**

Rationale: It is important to understand what the term means—to discriminate between mortality and survival.

28. Refer to Figure 10–2. From the information given regarding lung cancer in Figure 10–2, it can be determined that
   A. the incidence rate among black Americans is lower than that among white Americans.
   B. more white Americans are diagnosed with localized disease than black Americans.
   C. more black persons than white persons die of localized disease.
   D. among those diagnosed with localized disease, white persons have a better chance than black persons of surviving five years.

29. Refer to Figure 10–2. What are the five-year survival rates for cancers of the colon and rectum (all stages) for white and black persons, respectively, from 1974–1986?
   A. 54% and 46%, respectively.
   B. 6% and 5%, respectively.
   C. 85% and 55%, respectively.
   D. 52% and 16%, respectively.

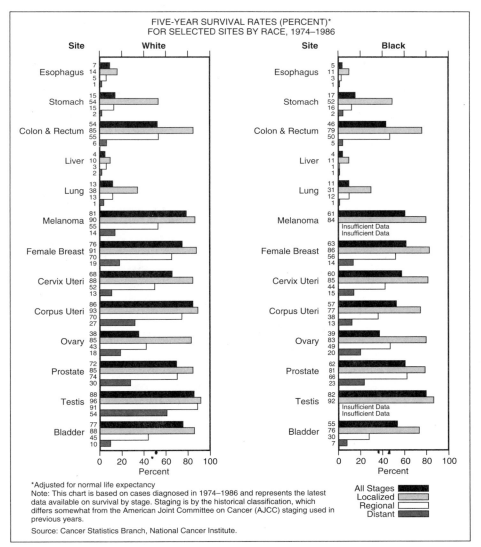

FIGURE 10–2. Five-year survival rates (percent)* for selected sites by race, 1974–1986. (Redrawn from Cancer Statistics Branch, National Cancer Institute, in, Boring CC, Squires TS, *Cancer Statistics, 1991. CA.* 41 (1): 21.

28. *Answer:* **D**

Rationale: Responses A, B, and C are wrong because the chart does not describe incidences or compare numbers of blacks to whites. It compares each group to itself with respect to survival rate, site, and stage. Response D is correct because information on the graph shows a 38% survival rate for whites versus a 31% survival rate for blacks.

29. *Answer:* **A**

Rationale: This question tests one's ability to correctly read and interpret graphic information.

30. Refer to Figure 10–2. From this figure you can determine
 A. the number of fatal cases of localized melanoma diagnosed in Americans from 1974–1986.
 B. the fatality rate for localized breast cancer in black females from 1974–1986.
 C. the number of black persons who survived for five years after being diagnosed with stomach cancer (all stages) from 1974–1986.
 D. the percentage of white females surviving five years after being diagnosed with localized breast cancer from 1974–1986.

31. From 1976-1986, gains in cancer survival occurred
 A. equally in black and white Americans, but less frequently among Hispanic Americans.
 B. more frequently in black than in white Americans.
 C. more frequently in white than in black Americans.
 D. equally among all races.

32. Significant gains in cancer survival in white Americans have occurred for all of the following sites **EXCEPT**
 A. testis.
 B. prostate.
 C. female breast.
 D. uterine cervix.

33. Which one of the following risk factors is responsible for the leading cause of cancer deaths in females in the United States?
 A. Multiple sexual partners.
 B. Smoking cigarettes.

 C. The "typical American diet"—low in fiber, high in fat.
 D. Excessive sunbathing.

34. Overall, women have a higher incidence of cancer than men, yet men have a higher incidence rate. The explanation for this is that
 A. the population of women is larger than the population of men.
 B. women have higher rates of gynecologic cancers than men have rates of genitourinary (e.g., prostate and testis) cancers.
 C. breast cancer artificially inflates the overall incidence of cancer in women.
 D. men have more occult malignancies.

35. For which of the following sites is the historic male/female "gender gap" in occurrence narrowing?
 A. Breast.
 B. Lung.
 C. Colon.
 D. Rectum.

36. Which of the following risk factors for cancer is least likely to be associated with socioeconomic status?
 A. Diet.
 B. Cigarette smoking.
 C. Sexual behavior.
 D. Family history of cancer.

37. High levels of cancer incidence and mortality in persons of lower socioeconomic status are most likely related to
 A. access to health care.
 B. genetic predispositions of different racial groups.
 C. differences in family functioning.
 D. level of formal education.

30. *Answer:* **D**

   Rationale: The graph does not describe fatal cases or fatality rates. It states the survival rate as a percentage, not the number of survivors.

31. *Answer:* **C**

   Rationale: Unequitable survival rates and trends between races are major problems in cancer epidemiology.

32. *Answer:* **D**

   Rationale: The increased survival rate for cancer of the uterine cervix has been minimal, 65 per 100,000 at five years if diagnosed in 1973 versus 67.8% per 100,000 if diagnosed in 1981.

33. *Answer:* **B**

   Rationale: Lung cancer is the leading cause of cancer deaths in females in the U.S., and the majority of these deaths are caused by smoking. Smoking is a lifestyle risk factor.

34. *Answer:* **A**

   Rationale: The key to answering this question correctly is carefully reading the stem. It differentiates between incidence (actual number of new cases) and incidence rate (actual number of new cases per the population at risk).

35. *Answer:* **B**

   Rationale: Smoking and lung cancer are important public health problems.

36. *Answer:* **D**

   Rationale: Family history of cancer suggests genetic predisposition rather than environmental effects.

37. *Answer:* **A**

   Rationale: Lack of access to health care is a major public health problem, particularly for the cancers amenable to secondary prevention (and primary prevention to a lesser extent). Response B occurs independently of socioeconomic status (SES); responses C and D are related to SES but not to cancer occurrence.

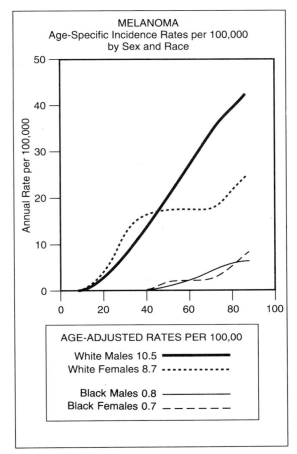

FIGURE 10–3. Age-specific incidence rates for melanoma per 100,000 individuals by sex and race. (Redrawn from Cancer Statistics Branch, National Cancer Institute, in, Boring CC, Squires TS. *Cancer Statistics, 1991. CA*. 41 (1): 21.

38. Refer to Figure 10–3. Which of the following statements is **NOT TRUE** based on Figure 10–3?
   A. Melanoma is much more common in whites than in blacks.
   B. The overall rates for black men and women are similar.
   C. In whites, rates are higher among women until age 50, when the rates for males increase.
   D. The rates for blacks are low throughout their life.

39. Statistics show that, with race as a discriminator, testicular cancer occurs
   A. more frequently in white males than in black males.
   B. more frequently in black males than in white males.
   C. equally in both races.
   D. more frequently in black males aged 15–35 than in white males.

40. Statistics show that, with race as a discriminator, prostate cancer occurs
   A. equally among black and white males.
   B. more frequently in black males than white males.
   C. more frequently in white males than black males.
   D. more frequently in white males under 50 years of age.

41. Which one of the following groups has the highest incidence and mortality rate for all cancers combined in the U.S.?
   A. African Americans.
   B. Hispanic Americans.
   C. Asian Americans.
   D. Caucasians.

42. In the United States, esophageal cancer is most common in which group?
   A. Native Americans.
   B. Blacks.
   C. Caucasians.
   D. Eastern Europeans.

43. Which one of the following cancers peaks in incidence in very young children (<5 years old), declines, then rises again steadily after age 30?
   A. Hodgkin's lymphoma.
   B. Leukemia.
   C. Wilm's tumor.
   D. Retinoblastoma.

38. *Answer:* **C**

Rationale: This question tests one's ability to accurately interpret common cancer graphs published by the ACS and National Cancer Institute.

39. *Answer:* **A**

Rationale: Testicular cancer is extremely rare in black men.

40. *Answer:* **B**

Rationale: Prostate cancer is an important public health problem that affects more black than white males in all age groups.

41. *Answer:* **A**

Rationale: African Americans have the highest incidence and mortality of all racial/ethnic groups in the U.S., and nurses need to be aware of this fact in terms of identification of high-risk groups. The relationship may relate more to socioeconomic status than to race, but at the present time, research has not established which is more important.

42. *Answer:* **B**

Rationale: Esophageal cancer is more common in blacks than in the other groups listed.

43. *Answer:* **B**

Rationale: The leukemias (all) peak at 6.6 per 100,000 below age 5, then decline until age 30, when they rise steadily to a high of 89.6 per 100,000 beyond age 85.

44. An adult between the ages of 65 and 79 is at highest risk of developing
    A. lung and bronchial cancer.
    B. colon cancer.
    C. urinary bladder cancer.
    D. chronic leukemia.

45. Which one of the following cancers peaks in incidence in young adulthood, declines, then rises again in old age?
    A. Testicular cancer in males.
    B. Breast cancer in females.
    C. Hodgkin's lymphoma in both sexes.
    D. Acute leukemia.

46. The occurrence of which cancer is virtually unheard of prior to age 40 in males, then rises with advancing age to a high of over 1100 per 100,000 at age 85 and over?
    A. Lung.
    B. Prostate.

    C. Testis.
    D. Lymphoma.

47. In general, the incidence of cancer related to age demonstrates
    A. peaks and valleys as one ages.
    B. a highest point in persons over 60.
    C. an increase at the beginning of each decade.
    D. a generally sharp and steady increase with age.

48. Which of the following is the single greatest risk factor for developing cancer?
    A. Advancing age.
    B. Female gender.
    C. Black race.
    D. Unhealthy lifestyle.

44. *Answer:* **A**

Rationale: Lung and bronchial cancer have the highest incidence beyond age 65 until age 80, when they begin to decline, and colon cancer incidence continues to rise.

45. *Answer:* **C**

Rationale: The incidence of Hodgkin's lymphoma reaches a high of 5.2 per 100,000 at age 20–24, then declines until age 45–49 (2.4 per 100,000), then rises steadily to 4.5 per 100,000 at age 80–84.

46. *Answer:* **B**

Rationale: This is the occurrence pattern of prostatic cancer.

47. *Answer:* **D**

Rationale: Cancer is more likely to occur as one ages.

48. *Answer:* **A**

Rationale: Cancer incidence rises exponentially with age.

REFERENCES

Boring CC, Squires TS, Tong T, (1991). Cancer Statistics. *CA*. 41: 19–51.

Cancer Statistics Review 1973–1987, (1990). Bethesda, MD: National Cancer Institute, Division of Cancer Prevention and Control Surveillance Program. U.S. Dept. of Health and Human Services, Public Health Service, National Institutes of Health. NIH Publication No. 90–2789.

Dangel RB, (1992). Cancer Epidemiology, in, Clark JC, McGee RF, (eds). *Core Curriculum for Oncology Nursing*, (2nd ed). Philadelphia: WB Saunders.

Frank-Stromborg M, (1991). Evaluating Cancer Risk, in, Baird SB, McCorkle R, Grant M, (eds). *Cancer Nursing. A Comprehensive Textbook*. Philadelphia, PA: WB Saunders, pp. 155–189.

Frank-Stromborg M, Cohen R, (1990). Assessment and Interventions for Cancer Prevention and Detection, in, Groenwald SL, Frogge MH, Goodman M, Yarbro CH, (eds). *Cancer Nursing Principles and Practice*, (2nd ed). Boston: Jones and Bartlett, pp. 119–160.

Mausner JS, Kramer S, (1985). *Epidemiology—An Introductory Text*. Philadelphia: WB Saunders.

Newell GR, (1985). Epidemiology of Cancer, in, DeVita VT, Hellman S, Rosenberg S, (eds). *Cancer Principles and Practice of Oncology*. Philadelphia: JB Lippincott, pp. 152–196.

Oleske DM, (1991). Epidemiologic Principles for Nursing Practice: Assessing the Cancer Problem and Planning Its Control, in, Baird SB, McCorkle R, Grant M, (eds). *Cancer Nursing: A Comprehensive Textbook*. Philadephia: WB Saunders, pp. 104–114.

Rosenberg JC, Lichter A, Leichman L, (1989). Cancer of the Esophagus, in, DeVita VT, Hellman S, Rosenberg S, (eds). *Cancer Principles and Practice of Oncology*, (3rd ed). Philadelphia: JB Lippincott, pp. 725–764.

11
Treatment of Cancer

Surgery
Thomas J. Szopa, Cathy L. Grace-Louthen

Radiation
Jennifer Dunn Bucholtz

Chemotherapy
Catherine M. Bender and Linda Tenenbaum

Biological Response Modifiers
Janice Beschorner and Marilyn Davis

Bone Marrow Transplantation
Kathy Coyle

Unproven Methods
Nancy E. Kane

Supportive Therapies and Procedures
Lynn Erdman, Marcia E. Rostad, and Leslie B. Tyson

Surgery
Thomas J. Szopa
Cathy L. Grace-Louthen

Select the BEST answer for all of the following questions:

1. Mrs. S had a local recurrence of breast cancer. She underwent a modified radical mastectomy. Such surgical therapy would be classified as
   A. definitive therapy.
   B. salvage therapy.
   C. palliative therapy.
   D. ablative therapy.

2. Mrs. H was scheduled for external beam-radiation therapy and radioactive breast implant. Such therapy would be referred to as
   A. definitive therapy.
   B. salvage therapy.
   C. ablative therapy.
   D. photodynamic therapy.

1. *Answer:* **B**

   Rationale: Surgery after local recurrence is considered salvage therapy because the patient has failed first-line therapy. Surgery may remove all disease locally. Salvage mastectomy results in a five-year survival rate of 50% when there is local recurrence of the disease.

2. *Answer:* **A**

   Rationale: Radiation is a form of local therapy. The use of external irradiation plus implantation has good results in local disease and a low incidence of radiation-induced toxicities.

3. Surgery is an effective and appropriate primary treatment for some cancers because
A. surgery can provide eradication of the disease locally as well as systemically.
B. cancers with a long cell cycle tend to be more locally confined.
C. cancers with a short cell cycle tend to be more locally confined.
D. surgery can provide eradication of the disease with the least amount of side effects.

4. Surgical excision performed to decrease local and systemic spread of the disease includes all of the following **EXCEPT**
A. use of a "no touch" technique consisting of frequent glove and instrument changes.
B. removal of tumor tissue with a wide margin of normal tissue.
C. removal of tumor tissue only up to the tumor margins.
D. ligation of draining lymphatics and blood vessels.

5. All of the following are true of laser therapy **EXCEPT** that it
A. precisely removes all cancer cells locally with maximum normal tissue preservation.
B. simultaneously seals off all blood vessels and lymphatics decreasing blood loss and dissemination of cancer cells.
C. is an easy delivery with minimal preparation required.
D. causes increased thermal tissue damage and, therefore, causes the same or increased functional disability compared to traditional surgery.

6. Photodynamic therapy is defined as
A. the intravenous injection of a light-sensitizing agent that is retained by tumor tissue, followed by exposure to laser, causing cytotoxicity.
B. a surgical procedure performed for the implantation of radioactive substances.

C. the endoscopic delivery of laser therapy.
D. a surgical method of intraoperative radiation therapy delivery.

7. Disadvantages of adjuvant therapy can include an increase of the type and severity of side effects from all therapies delivered. Some intra- and postoperative complications observed following adjuvant therapy include all of the following **EXCEPT**
A. delayed wound healing with some chemotherapeutic agents and laser therapy.
B. compromised respiratory functioning with lung irradiation and some chemotherapeutic agents.
C. compromised renal functioning with irradiation and some chemotherapeutic agents.
D. increased risk of cardiomyopathy with mediastinal irradiation and anthracycline therapy.

8. Other cancer treatment modalities are commonly used in conjunction with surgery. Adjuvant therapy
A. improves tumor resectability and alters the extent of surgery needed.
B. alters the extent of surgery needed but increases the functional disabilities following therapy.
C. provides more appealing options to patients but decreases treatment outcomes.
D. improves treatment outcomes but increases the functional disabilities following therapy.

9. Prophylactic cancer surgery is defined as
A. the reconstruction of anatomic defects created by cancer surgery to improve function and cosmetic appearance.
B. surgery performed on nonvital organs that have an extremely high incidence of subsequent cancer.
C. the insertion of various therapeutic hardware during active treatment periods to facilitate the delivery of treatment and increase patient comfort.
D. the removal of hormonal influence.

3. *Answer:* **B**

    Rationale: Surgery is an appropriate primary treatment for cancers with a long cell cycle time because they tend to be locally confined.

4. *Answer:* **C**

    Rationale: Tumors are resected with wide margins of normal tissue to increase the chances of complete removal of all malignant cells. This decreases potential for local and systemic spread of disease.

5. *Answer:* **D**

    Rationale: Responses A, B, and C describe the actions and advantages of laser therapy. Response D is a false statement.

6. *Answer:* **A**

    Rationale: This is the definition of photodynamic therapy.

7. *Answer:* **A**

    Rationale: Delayed wound healing is an effect of radiation therapy to a surgical site. Responses B, C, and D describe side effects of some combinations of therapy. Laser therapy does not delay wound healing.

8. *Answer:* **A**

    Rationale: Surgery is often used to remove as much of a tumor as possible. Adjuvant therapy reduces the tumor burden and increases the potential effectiveness of chemotherapy or radiation therapy while altering the extent of surgery needed.

9. *Answer:* **B**

    Rationale: Surgical removal of nonvital benign tissue or of an organ that is responsible for predisposing an individual to a high risk of cancer can lower the incidence and possibly prevent the occurrence of cancer.

10.   Mrs. C had an excisional biopsy performed on her left breast and a left axillary node dissection. An excisional biopsy means that Mrs. C
    A.   had a portion of tissue removed at the tumor margin for examination.
    B.   had an aspiration of fluid or tissue via a needle.
    C.   had the complete removal of the tumor with little or no margin of surrounding normal tissue removed.
    D.   had a large portion of her breast, which included the tumor, removed.

11.   The purpose of an excisional biopsy is to
    A.   establish tissue diagnosis and definitive treatment.
    B.   establish tissue diagnosis and determine surgical stage of disease.
    C.   establish tissue diagnosis and prophylactic surgery.
    D.   establish tissue diagnosis only.

12.   Which post-op activity decreases the incidence of infections?
    A.   Bed rest.
    B.   Early ambulation.
    C.   Placement of indwelling catheters.
    D.   Fluid restrictions.

13.   First-line treatment for cutaneous melanoma is
    A.   chemotherapy.
    B.   biological therapy.
    C.   surgical excision.
    D.   radiation therapy.

14.   Mr. J had a wide excision and groin dissection for synovial cell sarcoma. He calls your outpatient department, complaining of swelling, redness at the incision site, and a low-grade fever. You tell Mr. J,
    A.   "These symptoms are post-op symptoms."
    B.   "Take your antidiuretic medication."
    C.   "Call me if your fever increases, otherwise do nothing at present."
    D.   "You must come in to see the physician."

15.   Mr. S has undergone a radical head and neck dissection. In the postoperative period, he is placed in a semi-Fowler's position to
    A.   reduce facial edema.
    B.   facilitate respirations.
    C.   promote mucous drainage.
    D.   all of the above.

16.   Second-look surgical procedures are done for all of the following reasons **EXCEPT**
    A.   to check cancers that have the risk of local recurrence.
    B.   to check for residual disease.
    C.   to assess response to chemotherapy and/or radiation therapy.
    D.   to check the results of tumor markers.

17.   The definition of a wide excision or "en bloc" dissection is
    A.   removal of a wedge of tissue from a larger tumor mass.
    B.   obtaining a core of tissue through a needle.
    C.   removal of tumor, any tissues containing primary nodal drainage area, and any involved contiguous structures.
    D.   excision of the entire suspected lesion.

18.   A 4-year-old boy has cryptorchidism. Surgery is planned to repair this problem. What kind of surgical treatment is this?
    A.   Definitive.
    B.   Preventative.
    C.   Reconstructive.
    D.   Palliative.

19.   Cytoreductive therapy is considered the same as which treatment?
    A.   Adjuvant.
    B.   Debulking.
    C.   Definitive.
    D.   Palliative.

10. *Answer:* **C**

Rationale: Excisional therapy is used on small, accessible tumors. The entire mass is removed with little or no margin of surrounding normal tissue. In some cases, excisional biopsy alone is definitive therapy.

11. *Answer:* **A**

Rationale: Excisional therapy removes the entire tumor mass and is, therefore, definitive therapy. The purpose of all biopsies is to establish tissue diagnosis.

12. *Answer:* **B**

Rationale: Poor ventilation can account for significant numbers of infections. The urinary tract is often the source of sepsis. Avoiding post-op catheterization is important. Fluid restrictions do not have a role in the prevention of infections.

13. *Answer:* **C**

Rationale: Surgical treatment using a wide excision technique is the best option for cure.

14. *Answer:* **D**

Rationale: Infection is a potential post-op problem. The patient may be developing lymphedema or may need an antibiotic. The incisional site must be assessed by a physician.

15. *Answer:* **D**

Rationale: All of the above are appropriate to prevent postoperative complications.

16. *Answer:* **D**

Rationale: Second-look surgeries are less frequently done because blood tests (e.g., tumor markers and other diagnostic tests) provide information about tumor response.

17. *Answer:* **C**

Rationale: Response A is an incisional biopsy. Response B is a needle biopsy. Response D is an excisional biopsy.

18. *Answer:* **B**

Rationale: Because cryptorchidism is associated with the development of testicular cancer, orchiopexy is recommended before the age of 6. This is considered preventative surgery.

19. *Answer:* **B**

Rationale: Surgery may be done to debulk the tumor. This is called cytoreduction therapy.

REFERENCES

Aronoff B, (1986). The State of the Art in General Surgery and Surgical Oncology. *Laser Surgery and Medicine.* 6 (4): 376–382.

Dixon J, (1988). Current Laser Applications in General Surgery. *Annals of Surgery.* 207 (4): 355–372.

Frogge MH, Goodman M, (1990). Surgical Therapy, in, Groenwald SL, Frogge MH, Goodman M, Yarbro CH, (eds). *Cancer Nursing Principles and Practice,* (2nd ed). Boston: Jones and Bartlett, pp. 189–198.

Havard CP, Topping AE, (1991). Surgical Oncology, in, Baird SB, McCorkle R, Grant M, (eds). *Cancer Nursing: A Comprehensive Textbook.* Philadephia: WB Saunders, pp. 235–245.

Jako G, (1987). The Road Toward 21st Century Surgery: New Strategies and Initiatives in Cancer Treatment. *Laser Surgery and Medicine.* 7 (3): 217–218.

McClay E, et al., (1987). Preoperative Evaluation of the Oncology Patient. *Medical Clinics of North America.* 71 (3): 529–540.

Miaskowski C, (1991). Knowledge Deficit Related to Surgery, in, McNally JC, Somerville ET, Miaskowski C, Rostad M, (eds). *Guidelines for Oncology Nursing Practice,* (2nd ed). Philadelphia: WB Saunders, pp. 80–84.

——— (1987). Progress Symposium—Advances in Surgical Oncology. *World Journal of Surgery.* 11 (4): 405–540.

Rosenberg S, (1989). Principles of Surgical Oncology, in, DeVita VT, Hellman S, Rosenberg S, (eds). *Cancer Principles and Practice of Oncology,* (3rd ed). Philadelphia: JB Lippincott, pp. 236–246.

Shaneberger R, (1985). Effect of Chemotherapy and Radiotherapy on Wound Healing: Experimental Studies. *Recent Results Cancer Research.* 98: 17–34.

Szoya T, (1992). Implications of Surgical Treatment for Nursing, in, Clark JC, McGee RF, (eds). *Core Curriculum for Oncology Nursing,* (2nd ed). Philadelphia: WB Saunders.

Radiation

Jennifer Dunn Bucholtz

Select the BEST answer for all of the following questions.

1. Which of the following **BEST** describes the use of radiation therapy?
    A. Used in less than 25% of all persons with cancer.
    B. Generally considered a localized therapy.
    C. Generally considered a systemic therapy.
    D. Used only for malignant tumors.

2. Tumors comprised of predominantly _____ _____ cells are the most vulnerable to the effects of radiation therapy.
    A. poorly oxygenated
    B. undifferentiated
    C. dysplastic
    D. well-differentiated

3. Which of the following responses **BEST** describes the mechanism of action of ionizing radiation on living cells and tissues?
    A. Burning of the cell's nuclei.
    B. Bonding of the cell's water molecules.
    C. Alteration of the cell's RNA.
    D. Alteration of the cell's DNA.

4. Which of the following **BEST** describes an external beam radiation therapy treatment experience?
    A. An individual lies on a hard x-ray table alone in a fixed position.
    B. An individual lies on a hard x-ray table with a technologist in the room at all times.
    C. An individual lies on a hard x-ray table and senses heat in the area of the body being treated.
    D. An individual lies on a hard x-ray table that is moving during the actual treatment.

5. Which of the following responses **BEST** describes the purpose of simulation or radiation therapy treatment planning?
    A. To determine which type of radiation machine should be used.
    B. To determine the dosage of radiation to be given to the individual's tumor.
    C. To determine the number of treatments to be given to the individual's tumor.
    D. To determine the treatment field for the tumor volume.

6. Tumors that have a **HIGH** sensitivity to ionizing radiation include
    A. astrocytoma, seminoma, and salivary gland tumors.
    B. renal cancer, leukemia, and hepatoma.
    C. rhabdomyosarcoma, lymphoma, and chondrosarcoma.
    D. lymphoma, seminoma, and dysgerminoma.

7. Which of the following oncologic emergencies is **NOT** commonly treated with radiation therapy?
    A. Superior vena cava syndrome.
    B. Tumor lysis syndrome.
    C. Brain metastasis.
    D. Spinal cord compression.

8. Which of the following normal tissues are the **MOST** sensitive to ionizing radiation?
    A. Stomach, liver, and kidney.
    B. Lung, spinal cord, and small intestine.
    C. Heart, brain, and bone.
    D. Bone marrow, ovaries, and testes.

1. *Answer:* **B**

    Rationale: Radiation therapy is a localized treatment modality. Radiation is used in over 50% of all persons with cancer. Radiation is used to treat several benign conditions and tumors such as pituitary adenomas, desmoid tumors, and hyperthyroidism.

2. *Answer:* **B**

    Rationale: Undifferentiated cells tend to divide more frequently than well-differentiated cells. A cell is most radiosensitive when undergoing mitosis. Poorly oxygenated cells are relatively radioresistant. Dysplasia refers to an alteration in cell size, shape, and organization—none of which render a cell more or less radiosensitive.

3. *Answer:* **D**

    Rationale: Ionizing radiation kills cells by altering their DNA molecules.

4. *Answer:* **A**

    Rationale: The individual is alone when the actual treatment is given. He or she senses no heat. The treatment machine may be moving in some treatment setups, but not the table.

5. *Answer:* **D**

    Rationale: Both the dosage and the number of treatments are determined based on the type of tumor, size, stage, etc. Simulation is not used for these reasons. The type of radiation is chosen based on the individual's tumor depth and body size, or can be chosen based on scans and observation.

6. *Answer:* **D**

    Rationale: Lymphoma, seminoma, and dysgerminoma are all highly sensitive to radiation. All other tumors mentioned have a low or medium sensitivity.

7. *Answer:* **B**

    Rationale: Persons who have tumors that infiltrate the kidney may require radiation therapy to reduce the overall tumor burden. Chemotherapy may lead to tumor lysis syndrome. Tumor lysis syndrome is usually treated prophylactically with allopurinol and the regulation of renal function and metabolic status. With a very high white blood cell count (100,000), leukapheresis or dialysis may be needed.

8. *Answer:* **D**

    Rationale: The bone marrow, ovaries, and testes contain cells with rapid duplication times. These are the most sensitive cells based on the maximal tolerance dosage data for normal cells.

9. A patient who has been discharged from the hospital following removal of a cesium-137 gynecologic implant for cancer of the cervix calls her primary nurse complaining of diarrhea. Her primary nurse should advise her to
   A. take her antidiarrheal medication as prescribed.
   B. save her stools in a special container.
   C. increase her fluid intake and follow a high-protein, high-residue diet.
   D. return immediately to the hospital, because her stools are radioactive.

10. Examples of particle radiation used in radiation therapy treatments include
   A. alpha, beta, and gamma.
   B. alpha, beta, and x-rays.
   C. pions, neutrons, and beta.
   D. x-rays, beta, and gamma.

11. Sources of gamma radiation used in radiation treatments include
   A. yttrium-90, iridium-192, and iodine-131.
   B. strontium-90, radium-226, and phosphorus-32.
   C. iodine-131, iridium-192, and radium-226.
   D. cobalt-60, iodine-131, and phosphorus-32.

12. A 68-year-old man who is receiving external radiation therapy to the brain after a craniotomy for a glioblastoma multiform complains of pain in his right calf. He asks his nurse if this pain can, in any way, be caused by the radiation therapy. His nurse answers:
   A. the cranial radiation may be the cause of his calf pain.
   B. the cranial radiation is not the cause of his calf pain.
   C. the calf pain may represent bone metastasis.
   D. the calf pain may be from the effects of internal radiation.

13. Which of the following responses **BEST** explains the rationale for combining hyperthermia with radiation therapy?
   A. Hyperthermia and radiation both kill cells in the dividing phase of the cell cycle and have an **ADDITIVE** effect.
   B. Hyperthermia kills cells in a resting phase, and radiation kills cells in a dividing phase; they have a **SYNERGISTIC** effect.
   C. Hyperthermia and radiation both work best in the presence of oxygen and have a **SYNERGISTIC** effect.
   D. Hyperthermia and radiation work best in divided doses and have an **ADDITIVE** effect.

14. Which of the following **BEST** explains why children may experience long-term side effects different from adults when treated with radiation therapy to the same body tissues?
   A. Children are given higher radiation doses than adults for the same tumors.
   B. Children are better able to tolerate ionizing radiation.
   C. Children's developing tissues are more radioresistant than an adult's fully developed tissues.
   D. Children's developing tissues are more sensitive to radiation damage than an adult's fully developed tissues.

15. Which of the following **BEST** explains why radiation therapy treatments are given in divided or fractionated doses over a period of time?
   A. One radiation treatment would be too expensive.
   B. Radiation machines cannot deliver large doses at one time.
   C. Tumor cells are better killed with small doses of radiation given over time.
   D. Normal cells can better tolerate small doses of radiation.

9. *Answer:* **A**

Rationale: Patients who have a sealed source of cesium-137 in place are not radioactive, nor are their body fluids. Patients who are experiencing diarrhea should be advised to follow a low-residue diet.

10. *Answer:* **C**

Rationale: Gamma and x-rays are electromagnetic sources. Alpha radiation is not specifically used for treatment purposes.

11. *Answer:* **C**

Rationale: Phosphorus-32, yttrium-90, and strontium-90 are pure beta emitters. All of the others are sources of gamma radiation.

12. *Answer:* **B**

Rationale: Radiation to the brain will not cause calf pain. There are no systemic radiation effects resulting from brain radiation. In this situation, it is possible that the man has a blood clot in his leg related to the diagnosis and surgery.

13. *Answer:* **B**

Rationale: The actions of hyperthermia and radiation are synergistic. Hyperthermia kills cells in a resting phase and kills hypoxic cells. Radiation therapy kills cells in a dividing phase.

14. *Answer:* **D**

Rationale: Developing tissues are much more sensitive to radiation damage. Children who have active developing tissues treated have the risk of more long-term side effects than adults. Children under the age of 6, for example, may show cognitive changes, after radiation to the brain, which are not seen in adults treated with radiation to the brain.

15. *Answer:* **D**

Rationale: Radiation therapy doses are fractionated so that normal cells can repair themselves between daily fractions. Radiation therapy machines can be programmed to deliver any specified dose. The cost is not an issue in fractionation.

16.   When planning radiation safety measures for a particular procedure, the **MOST IMPORTANT** factors a nurse should inquire about are
    A.   the radioisotope's half-life, length of use, and cost.
    B.   the type of radiation emitted, half-life, and patient compliance.
    C.   the type of radiation emitted, radiation monitoring, and cost of the isotope.
    D.   the type of radiation emitted, amount of isotope, half-life, and method of isotope delivery.

17.   A 42-year-old woman is given 100 millicuries of oral radioactive iodine-131 for thyroid cancer. Once the radioisotope is swallowed, which of the following instructions should **NOT** be given?
    A.   She can be out of bed inside her room.
    B.   She can leave her room for one hour per day.
    C.   She can use the bathroom facilities.
    D.   She must remain inside her room until she emits a specified, low amount of radioactivity.

18.   Which of the following **BEST** lists the possible side effects of a full course of external beam-radiation therapy to the mediastinum?
    A.   Dry mouth, skin reaction, and nausea.
    B.   Esophagitis, nausea, and headache.
    C.   Nausea, skin reaction, and myocardial infarct.
    D.   Esophagitis, fatigue, and skin reaction.

19.   Which of the following responses **BEST** explains why a woman with cancer of the cervix should perform vaginal dilation following a curative treatment with external radiation and a radiation implant?
    A.   Prevention of vaginal infections.
    B.   Prevention of difficult vaginal delivery.
    C.   Prevention of tumor recurrence.
    D.   Prevention of vaginal tightening and fibrosis.

20.   The area of the body most likely to lead to bone marrow depression when treated with radiation is the
    A.   brain.
    B.   head and neck.
    C.   breast.
    D.   pelvis.

21.   Which of the following responses **BEST** describes the purpose of using lead blocks during radiation therapy?
    A.   To make the shape of the radiation beam a square or rectangle.
    B.   To keep radiation from scattering inside the body.
    C.   To keep radiation from penetrating to certain normal tissues.
    D.   To keep the radiation dose to a minimum.

22.   A 55-year-old woman receiving external beam-radiation to her left breast for stage I breast cancer complains of redness and soreness under her breast on the second day of treatment. Which of the following **BEST** describes what the nurse should do first?
    A.   Inspect the woman's skin.
    B.   Instruct the woman to apply zinc oxide to the skin under the breast that is red and sore.
    C.   Instruct the woman to keep her bra on during the remaining radiation treatments.
    D.   Instruct the woman to apply cool compresses to the irritated skin.

16. *Answer:* **D**

Rationale: The cost of the isotope has no bearing on safety measures. Although compliance is important, the type of radiation emitted, the amount of the isotope, and method of delivery are more important.

17. *Answer:* **B**

Rationale: With this amount of radioactive iodine-131, she must remain inside her room in radiation isolation until response D is met. Individuals who swallow this isotope can be out of bed and use the bathroom facilities, but should be behind a lead shield when someone enters the room.

18. *Answer:* **D**

Rationale: Esophagitis, fatigue, and skin reactions are all frequently observed side effects of mediastinal radiation. Individuals do not experience a dry mouth, headache, or myocardial infarct from mediastinal irradiation.

19. *Answer:* **D**

Rationale: Radiation will cause vaginal fibrosis and stenosis when full-dose curative therapy is given. Curative therapy will render the woman infertile. Vaginal dilation does not prevent infections or tumor recurrence.

20. *Answer:* **D**

Rationale: The pelvis contains a large amount of bone marrow.

21. *Answer:* **C**

Rationale: Custom lead blocks are made to protect normal tissues, thus shaping the beam to treat the desired tissues.

22. *Answer:* **A**

Rationale: Nursing intervention begins with inspection of the skin. It is unlikely that the red and sore skin is due to radiation effects after only two treatments. Responses B and D should not be advised because both will

increase the possibility of radiation skin reaction over time. Any clothing or dressings in the field of radiation will alter the absorption and distribution of the radiation.

REFERENCES

Brager BL, Yasko J, (1984). *Care of the Client Receiving Chemotherapy.* Reston, Va: Reston Publishing Co.

Buckoltz JD, (1992). Implications of Radiation Therapy for Nursing, in, Clark JC, McGee RF, (eds). *Core Curriculum for Oncology Nursing,* (2nd ed). Philadelphia: WB Saunders.

Dietz KA, Flaherty AM, (1990). Oncologic Emergencies, in, Groenwald SL, Frogge MH, Goodman M, Yarbro CH, (eds). *Cancer Nursing Principles and Practice,* (2nd ed). Boston: Jones and Bartlett, pp. 644–668.

Hilderly L, (1990). Radiotherapy, in, Groenwald SL, Frogge MH, Goodman M, Yarbro CH, (eds). *Cancer Nursing Principles and Practice,* (2nd ed). Boston: Jones and Bartlett, pp. 199–229.

Hilderley LJ, Daro KH, (1991). Radiation Oncology, in, Baird SB, McCorkle R, Grant M, (eds). *Cancer Nursing: A Comprehensive Textbook.* Philadephia: WB Saunders, pp. 246–265.

Hogan CM, (1991). Sexual Dysfunction Related to Disease Process and Treatment, in, McNally JC, Somerville CT, Miaskowski C, Rostad M, (eds). *Guidelines for Cancer Nursing Practice,* (2nd ed). Philadelphia: WB Saunders, pp. 339–344.

McNally JC, Strohl RA, (1991). Skin Integrity, Impairment of, Related to Radiation Therapy, in, McNally JC, Somerville ET, Miaskowski C, Rostad M, (eds). *Guidelines for Oncology Nursing Practice,* (2nd ed). Philadelphia: WB Saunders, pp. 236–240.

Sandland R, Barrett A, (1986). Radiation Therapy, in, Voute VA, et al. (eds). *Cancer in Children: Clinical Management.* New York: Springer Verlag, pp. 41.

Shell JA, (1992). Knowledge Deficit Related to Radiation Therapy, in, McNally JC, Somerville ET, Miaskowski C, Rostad M, (eds). *Guidelines for Oncology Nursing Practice,* (2nd ed). Philadelphia: WB Saunders, pp. 62–69.

Strohl RA, (1988). The Nursing Role in Radiation Oncology: Symptom Management of Acute and Chronic Reactions. *Oncology Nursing Forum.* 15 (4): 429–434.

Strohl RA, (1992). Knowledge Deficit Related to Brochytherapy (Implants), in, McNally JC, Somerville ET, Miaskowski C, Rostad M, (eds). *Guidelines for Oncology Nursing Practice,* (2nd ed). Philadelphia: WB Saunders, pp. 70–75.

Tannock IF, (1989). Principles of Cell Proliferation: Cell Kinetics, in, DeVita VT, Hellman S, Rosenberg S, (eds). *Cancer Principles and Practice of Oncology,* (3rd ed). Philadelphia: JB Lippincott, pp. 3–13.

Yasko J, (1982). *Care of the Client Receiving External Radiation Therapy.* Reston, VA: Reston Publishing Co.

Chemotherapy

Catherine M. Bender and Linda Tenenbaum

Select the BEST answer for all of the following questions:

1. By definition, the cell cycle
   A. is the process of cellular reproduction.
   B. consists of three phases.
   C. occurs only in malignant cells.
   D. is independent of cell type.

2. The most common route of chemotherapy administration is
   A. oral.
   B. intramuscular.
   C. intravenous.
   D. subcutaneous.

3. Combinations of chemotherapeutic agents are developed according to all of the following criteria **EXCEPT**:
   A. agents that possess differing dose-limiting toxicities.
   B. agents that affect different points in the cell cycle.
   C. agents that possess nadirs occurring at the same time points.
   D. agents whose combined effects produce enhanced cytotoxic effects over single agent therapy.

4. Which of the following are vesicant chemotherapeutic agents?
   A. Vincristine, vinblastine, and doxorubicin.
   B. Vincristine, bleomycin, and mechlorethamine.
   C. Cyclophosphamide, doxorubicin, and vincristine.
   D. Vincristine, mechlorethamine, and cyclophosphamide.

5. Cancer chemotherapy functions at the cellular level by
   A. interrupting the cell cycle.
   B. promoting the cell cycle.
   C. hastening the cell cycle.
   D. modifying the cell cycle.

6. Which of the following factors influence the success of treatment with chemotherapy?
   A. Mitotic rate of the cell type of the malignancy.
   B. Size of the tumor.
   C. Presence of chemotherapy-resistant cells.
   D. All of the above.

7. Cancer chemotherapeutic agents are classified according to their
   A. route of administration.
   B. mechanism of action.
   C. mode of preparation.
   D. degree of toxicity.

8. Antitumor antibiotics
   A. are cell cycle nonspecific agents.
   B. are cell cycle specific agents.
   C. inhibit RNA synthesis.
   D. are effective during mitosis.

9. The aim of adjuvant chemotherapy is to
   A. offset the existence of resistant cells.
   B. enable ease of chemotherapy administration.
   C. eradicate remaining micrometastases following primary treatment.
   D. palliate the symptoms of patients in whom cure is not possible.

10. Cardiac toxicity is most strongly associated with which of the following chemotherapy agents?
    A. Vincristine.
    B. Adriamycin.
    C. Nitrogen mustard.
    D. Cisplatinum.

1. *Answer:* **A**

    Rationale: The cell cycle is the sequential phase of cellular reproduction and occurs in all cells.

2. *Answer:* **C**

    Rationale: Most chemotherapy agents are unstable when given by mouth or by intramuscular or subcutaneous routes.

3. *Answer:* **C**

    Rationale: Responses A, B, and D are known characteristics of combination chemotherapy. Response C is incorrect because the nadir is a dose-limiting toxicity and agents are selected with different dose-limiting toxicities.

4. *Answer:* **A**

    Rationale: Vincristine, vinblastine, doxorubicin and mechlorethamine are vesicant agents; bleomycin and cyclophosphamide are not vesicant agents.

5. *Answer:* **A**

    Rationale: Chemotherapy causes interruptions in the cell cycle promoting tumor cell lysis.

6. *Answer:* **C**

    Rationale: Most active cytotoxic agents selectively target rapidly proliferating cells. A single dose of an agent kills a fraction of tumor cells. Tumors mutate spontaneously toward drug resistance.

7. *Answer:* **B**

    Rationale: Chemotherapeutic agents share drug similarities that allow these agents to be classified according to their mechanism of action.

8. *Answer:* **A**

    Rationale: Antitumor antibiotics are considered to be cell cycle nonspecific agents.

9. *Answer:* **C**

    Rationale: The use of adjuvant therapy after primary interventions, such as surgery, is aimed at controlling the malignancy by preventing recurrence.

10. *Answer:* **B**

    Rationale: Cardiotoxicity is the dose-limiting toxicity of adriamycin.

11.   Mr. W is a 61-year-old male who was treated with adriamycin postoperatively for a high grade sarcoma four years ago. Today, at work, he noticed increased fatigue, a nonproductive cough, and mild shortness of breath. He should be instructed by the company's health provider to
A.   go home and rest—he is overworked.
B.   take a longer lunch and return to work.
C.   call his private physician for an appointment.
D.   go directly to the nearest emergency room.

12.   Factors that increase the risk of cardiotoxicity secondary to treatment with adriamycin include all of the following **EXCEPT**
A.   advanced age.
B.   concurrent administration of cyclophosphamide.
C.   prior radiation to the mediastinum.
D.   prior immunotherapy.

13.   The dose-limiting toxicity in the administration of adriamycin is
A.   cardiotoxicity.
B.   bladder toxicity.
C.   hepatic toxicity.
D.   neurotoxicity.

14.   By definition, cell cycle nonspecific agents
A.   are effective against cells that are in cycle as well as those in the resting phase.
B.   exert their effects at any point during the cell cycle when cells are reproducing.
C.   are generally administered by continuous infusion.
D.   are only active during DNA synthesis.

15.   Intravesicular chemotherapy is administered
A.   via an Ommaya reservoir.
B.   directly into the central nervous system.
C.   into the bladder in high concentrations.
D.   systemically to distribute the chemotherapeutic agent.

16.   Cell cycle specific agents exert their major cytotoxic effects
A.   against cells that are in cycle as well as those that are in the resting phase.
B.   only against cells in the resting phase.
C.   during a specific phase in the cell cycle.
D.   none of the above.

17.   The rationale for using combinations of chemotherapeutic agents is that combinations
A.   potentially offset the existence of chemotherapy-resistant cells.
B.   include agents that are able to kill cells that are dividing as well as those that are resting.
C.   have the potential ability to produce improved cytotoxic effects over single agent therapy.
D.   all of the above.

18.   Which one of the following malignancies is possible to cure with chemotherapy as the primary mode of treatment?
A.   Colon cancer.
B.   Head and neck cancer.
C.   Hodgkin's disease.
D.   Lung cancer.

19.   Intraperitoneal chemotherapy
A.   produces more severe side effects than intravenous therapy.
B.   is palliative treatment.
C.   can only be administered via a Tenckhoff catheter.
D.   maximizes direct contact of tumor cells with the chemotherapeutic agent.

20.   All of the following are true statements about intrathecal/intraventricular administration of chemotherapy **EXCEPT**
A.   it delivers chemotherapy directly to the central nervous system.
B.   it can only be administered via lumbar puncture.
C.   it offsets the problem of the inability of most chemotherapeutic agents to pass the blood–brain barrier.
D.   it may be associated with complications such as headache, stiff neck, and seizures.

11. *Answer:* **D**

Rationale: These could be subtle signs and symptoms of cardiotoxicity and the clinical picture of congestive heart failure with his history of adriamycin administration. He needs immediate attention to assess his cardiac status.

12. *Answer:* **D**

Rationale: Immunotherapy is not known to increase the risk of cardiotoxicity. All of the other factors do. Identifying high-risk clients is an important aspect of early detection of cardiotoxicity.

13. *Answer:* **A**

Rationale: Cardiotoxicity is the dose-limiting side effect of adriamycin. The abnormalities range from apparently harmless, subtle EKG changes to life-threatening cardiomyopathy. It is recommended that the cumulative dosage of adriamycin not exceed 450 mg/m^2.

14. *Answer:* **A**

Rationale: Cell cycle nonspecific agents are active against cells in all phases of the cell cycle.

15. *Answer:* **C**

Rationale: Intravesicular refers to instillation of a substance into the bladder via a Foley catheter.

16. *Answer:* **C**

Rationale: Cell cycle specific agents exert their effect only during specific phases of cellular development.

17. *Answer:* **D**

Rationale: The rationale for combination chemotherapy includes all three components of sensitivity, decreased resistance, and greater cytotoxic effects on malignant cells in various phases of development.

18. *Answer:* **C**

Rationale: 85% of Hodgkin's disease is curable with chemotherapy as the primary mode of treatment.

19. *Answer:* **D**

Rationale: Intraperitoneal instillation of chemotherapy provides direct contact of the agent with cells in the peritoneal cavity.

20. *Answer:* **B**

Rationale: Intrathecal/intraventricular administration may be via an Ommaya reservoir.

21. Normal and malignant cells with high mitotic rates are
    A. more susceptible to the actions of chemotherapeutic agents.
    B. more responsive to agents in the S phase of the cell cycle.
    C. less susceptible to combination chemotherapy.
    D. less responsive to any chemotherapy.

22. In which phase are malignant as well as normal cells refractory to most cancer chemotherapy agents?
    A. G_0 phase.
    B. G_1 phase.
    C. S phase.
    D. Mitosis.

23. Which part of the cell cycle follows mitosis?
    A. The S phase.
    B. Cell division.
    C. Cell differentiation into immature cells.
    D. Cell maturation and replication.

24. By definition, mitosis is:
    A. the actual phase of cell division.
    B. responsible for DNA synthesis.
    C. the resting phase of the cell cycle.
    D. responsible for RNA and protein synthesis.

25. By definition, the S phase of the cell cycle is
    A. the resting phase.
    B. responsible for RNA and protein synthesis.
    C. the phase during which the mitotic spindle apparatus is produced.
    D. the phase during which DNA is synthesized.

26. By definition, the G_0 phase of the cell cycle is
    A. the actual phase of cell division.
    B. very consistent in terms of its length of time.
    C. the resting phase.
    D. the phase in which the cell is in the process of division.

27. The proper site for the intravenous administration of a vesicant chemotherapy agent is
    A. the metacarpal vein.
    B. any vein 1/2 to 1 inch above the wrist.
    C. any vein 1/2 to 1 inch below the antecubital region.
    D. any forearm vein at least 2 inches from the antecubital or wrist areas.

28. Body surface area (BSA) is the
    A. $\dfrac{\text{height} \times \text{weight}}{10}$
    B. muscle mass of an individual.
    C. basis for calculating chemotherapy dosage.
    D. $\dfrac{\text{weight}}{\text{height}}$

EG EG

21. *Answer:* **A**

Rationale: This principle underscores the rationale for the action of cancer chemotherapeutic agents, and also for the occurrence of side effects.

22. *Answer:* **A**

Rationale: G_0 is the resting phase of the cell cycle. No cell reproduction occurs in this phase.

23. *Answer:* **D**

Rationale: Following mitosis, cells mature and either enter G_1 to repeat the cell cycle or go to G_0 until triggered to reenter the cell cycle.

24. *Answer:* **A**

Rationale: Cell division occurs during mitosis.

25. *Answer:* **D**

Rationale: DNA is synthesized during the S phase of the cell cycle.

26. *Answer:* **C**

Rationale: G_0 is the resting, inactive phase of the cell cycle.

27. *Answer:* **D**

Rationale: Veins in the antecubital and wrist areas, and within 2 inches from those regions, should be avoided when administering a vesicant.

28. *Answer:* **C**

Rationale: BSA is used to determine the optimal chemotherapy dosage for each patient.

29.   Mrs. S's chemotherapy dose is to be calculated in mg/m^2. She weighs 130 pounds (59 kg) and is 5'3" (160 cm) tall. Using the nomogram in Figure 11–1, calculate Mrs. S's m^2.
    A.   1.42.
    B.   1.53.
    C.   1.59.
    D.   1.61.

30.   Long-term effects of exposure to cytotoxic agents are usually seen during which period following exposure?
    A.   Forty-eight to seventy-two hours.
    B.   Three to ten days.
    C.   Ten to thirty days.
    D.   Sixty days or more.

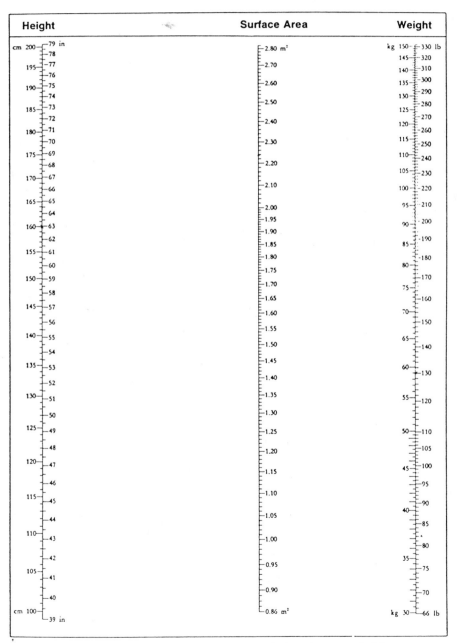

FIGURE 11–1. Nomogram for calculating the body surface area of adults.

29. *Answer:* **D**

Rationale: Nomograms, or body surface area calculators, are used to calculate chemotherapy dosage based on mg/m^2.

30. *Answer:* **D**

Rationale: The period for long-term effects is "months or years" after exposure. Sixty days or more relates to this time period.

31. Select the short-term effects of exposure to cytotoxic agents.
   A. Partial alopecia, chromosomal abnormalities, and dermatitis.
   B. Hyperpigmentation, partial alopecia, and chromosomal abnormalities.
   C. Dermatitis, partial alopecia, and headache.
   D. Dermatitis, hyperpigmentation, and headache.

32. A disposable, plastic-backed table pad in the area where chemotherapy drugs are prepared should be changed
   A. after each medication is prepared.
   B. when leaving the work area for a break.
   C. at the completion of each shift.
   D. after preparing vesicant medications.

33. Gloves used in preparing chemotherapy medications should have the following characteristics:
   A. disposable, surgical latex, long-cuffed, talc-free.
   B. disposable, polyvinyl chloride (PVC), long-cuffed, powdered.
   C. non-disposable, surgical latex, long-cuffed, talc-free.
   D. disposable, surgical latex, short-cuffed, powdered.

34. According to OSHA guidelines, the blower on the airflow hood of a biological safety cabinet should be on
   A. whenever medication is being prepared.
   B. when preparing medications that emit inhalable vapors.
   C. during and for two hours after chemotherapy preparation.
   D. twenty-four hours a day, seven days a week.

35. Needles and syringes used for chemotherapy preparation should be disposed of in containers that are
   A. surgical latex.
   B. puncture-resistant.
   C. sterile.
   D. biodegradable.

36. Emergency measures for accidental eye contact with a cytotoxic agent should include all of the following **EXCEPT**
   A. irrigating the eye(s) with isotonic solution for five minutes.
   B. having eye(s) examined by a physician.
   C. documenting the incident according to policy.
   D. reporting the incident to poison control.

37. The ONS Outcome Standards for Chemotherapy Administration were prepared to provide for
   A. safety to personnel, patients, and the environment.
   B. specific procedures for diluting and administering vesicant chemotherapeutic agents.
   C. steps to be followed when administering investigational chemotherapeutic agents.
   D. a mode of evaluating effectiveness of chemotherapeutic agents.

38. The nurse may be exposed to cytotoxic agents by all of the following routes **EXCEPT**
   A. absorption through skin.
   B. inhalation of aerosols.
   C. direct eye contact.
   D. extravasation of drugs.

39. Central venous administration of chemotherapy can be achieved via an
   A. implanted venous access device.
   B. Ommaya reservoir.
   C. Tenckhoff catheter.
   D. peripheral IV catheter.

40. All of the following describe intrapleural chemotherapy **EXCEPT** that
   A. it is administered via a thoracotomy tube.
   B. it is administered with the aim of sclerosing the pleural lining.
   C. it requires that the pleural cavity be drained as completely as possible prior to administration.
   D. it crosses the blood–brain barrier.

31. *Answer:* **D**

    Rationale: Dermatitis, hyperpigmentation, and headache are three short-term effects. Other choices each include one long-term effect.

32. *Answer:* **C**

    Rationale: OSHA guidelines recommend changing plastic-backed disposable pads at the completion of each shift.

33. *Answer:* **A**

    Rationale: The recommended composition and style of gloves, according to OSHA, ONS, and ASHP guidelines, is disposable, surgical latex, long-cuffed, and talc-free.

34. *Answer:* **D**

    Rationale: OSHA guideline specifications.

35. *Answer:* **B**

    Rationale: OSHA guideline specifications.

36. *Answer:* **D**

    Rationale: It is not necessary to report accidental eye contact to poison control. Immediate irrigation of the affected eye(s) must be done.

37. *Answer:* **A**

    Rationale: Stated in ONS Outcome Standards.

38. *Answer:* **D**

    Rationale: Extravasation is a patient exposure. Other responses are all modes of exposure of the nurse.

39. *Answer:* **A**

    Rationale: Implanted venous access device is the only method listed that provides direct access to the central vein.

40. *Answer:* **D**

    Rationale: Intrapleural access delivers chemotherapy to the pleural cavity.

41.   After an extravasation in the right lower arm, the client should be encouraged to use his or her right arm
   A.   as much as possible.
   B.   for light activity only for five to seven days.
   C.   after resting the extremity for forty-eight to seventy-two hours.
   D.   only if it is not painful during use.

42.   When extravasation of a vesicant is suspected, the first action of the nurse is to discontinue administration of the medication and
   A.   irrigate the IV with 5–10 ml saline.
   B.   remove the IV needle immediately.
   C.   attempt to aspirate residual medication.
   D.   apply pressure to the site.

43.   Cold may be applied to a chemotherapy extravasation site. This will achieve all of the following **EXCEPT**
   A.   facilitating dispersion of subcutaneous antidote.
   B.   decreasing the absorption of medication.
   C.   reducing the amount of drug that enters cells.
   D.   minimizing local pain.

44.   Local instillation of hyaluronidase is the manufacturer's recommended antidote for extravasation of
   A.   doxorubicin.
   B.   vincristine.
   C.   mechlorethamine.
   D.   busulfan.

45.   Heat is the initial recommended treatment for extravasation of
   A.   doxorubicin.
   B.   vincristine.
   C.   mechlorethamine.
   D.   busulfan.

46.   The nurse should be aware that extravasation of a vesicant chemotherapeutic agent will
   A.   be accompanied by some degree of pain.
   B.   present with a burning sensation as an early symptom.
   C.   be evident within ten minutes after completion of the medication administration.
   D.   develop in some instances with no pain or burning.

47.   Select the statement that *best* describes a vesicant and an irritant.
   A.   The term "vesicant" is used when referring to antineoplastic agents; irritant refers to other types of agents.
   B.   A vesicant commonly results in pain along the path of the vein; an irritant does not.
   C.   A vesicant has the potential to cause tissue destruction; an irritant does not.
   D.   A vesicant cannot be given by IV push; an irritant can.

48.   The major activity of antimetabolites occurs during which phase of the cell cycle?
   A. G_0 phase.
   B. G_1 phase.
   C.   S phase.
   D.   M phase.

49.   Metacarpal veins are suitable for administration of
   A.   any intravenous chemotherapeutic agent.
   B.   medications prepared in dilute concentrations.
   C.   IV push medications only.
   D.   non-vesicant chemotherapeutic agents.

41. *Answer:* **A**

    Rationale: Use of the affected arm will aid in the reabsorption of extravasated medication and reduce the time required for healing.

42. *Answer:* **C**

    Rationale: Once the drug is stopped, aspiration of any residual medication is the initial intervention. The needle should not be irrigated or removed until it is ascertained whether an antidote is to be instilled.

43. *Answer:* **A**

    Rationale: Cold causes constriction of vessels, reducing the dispersion of the subcutaneous antidote.

44. *Answer:* **B**

    Rationale: Hyaluronidase is the manufacturer's recommendation for local treatment of extravasation of vincristine and other vinca alkaloids.

45. *Answer:* **B**

    Rationale: The manufacturers recommend application of heat for the treatment of extravasation of vincristine and other vinca alkaloids.

46. *Answer:* **D**

    Rationale: It is important for the nurse to recall that an extravasation of a vesicant chemotherapeutic agent can occur without symptoms of pain or burning.

47. *Answer:* **C**

    Rationale: C is the only response that properly describes both a vesicant and an irritant.

48. *Answer:* **C**

    Rationale: Antimetabolites affect DNA synthesis in the S phase of the cell cycle.

49. *Answer:* **D**

    Rationale: Metacarpal veins are NOT recommended for administration of vesicant medications.

REFERENCES

Brager BL, Yasko JM, (1984). *Care of the Client Receiving Chemotherapy*. Reston, VA: Reston Publishing Co.

Bender C, (1992). Implications of Antineoplastic Therapy for Nursing, in, Clark JC, McGee RF, (eds). *Core Curriculum for Oncology Nursing*, (2nd ed). Philadelphia: WB Saunders.

Cancer Chemotherapy Guidelines, (1988). Pittsburgh: Oncology Nursing Society.

Fischer DS, Knobf MT, (1989). *The Cancer Chemotherapy Handbook*, (3rd ed). Chicago: Year Book Medical Publishers Inc.

Fiscus JA, Hayes NA, Rostad ME, Whedon MA, (1989). *Safe Handling of Cytoxic Drugs, Independent Study Modules*. Pittsburgh: Oncology Nursing Society.

Goodman M, (1991). Delivery of Cancer Chemotherapy, in, Baird SB, McCorkle R, Grant M, (eds). *Cancer Nursing: A Comprehensive Textbook*. Philadephia: WB Saunders, pp. 291–320.

Goodman M, Stoner C, (1991). Mucous Membrane Integrity, Impairment of, Related to Stomatitis, in, McNally JC, Somerville CT, Miaskowski C, Rostad M, (eds). *Guidelines for Cancer Nursing Practice*, (2nd ed). Philadelphia: WB Saunders, pp. 241–247.

Hoff ST, (1987). Concepts in Intraperitoneal Chemotherapy. *Seminars in Oncology Nursing*. 3 (2): 112–117.

Legha SS, Hortobagy GN, Benjamin RS, (1987). Anthracyclines, in, Lokich JJ, (ed). *Cancer Chemotherapy by Infusion*. Chicago: Precept Press, pp. 130–144.

McNally JC, Stair J, (1991). Potential for Infection, in, McNally JC, Somerville ET, Miaskowski C, Rostad M, (eds). *Guidelines for Oncology Nursing Practice*, (2nd ed). Philadelphia: WB Saunders, pp. 191–202.

OSHA Instruction Publication 8-1.1, (1986). *Guidelines for Cytoxic (Antineoplastic Drugs)*. Washington DC: US Department of Labor, Jan. 29.

Skeel RT, (ed), (1982). *Manual of Cancer Chemotherapy*. Boston: Little, Brown Co.

Somerville ET, (1991). Knoweldge Deficit Related to Chemotherapy, in, McNally JC, Somerville ET, Miaskowski C, Rostad M, (eds). *Guidelines for Oncology Nursing Practice*, (2nd ed). Philadelphia: WB Saunders, pp. 57–61.

Tenenbaum L, (1989). *Cancer Chemotherapy: A Reference Guide*. Philadelphia: WB Saunders.

Tenenbaum L, (1992). Principles of Preparation, Administration and Disposal of Antineoplastic Agents, in, Clark JC, McGee RF, (eds). *Core Curriculum for Oncology Nursing*, (2nd ed). Philadelphia: WB Saunders.

Van Hoff D, Rozwnweig M, Piccart M, (1982). The Cardiotoxicity of Anticancer Agents. *Seminars in Oncology*. 9 (1): 23–33.

Biological Response Modifiers

Janice Beschorner
Marilyn Davis

Select the BEST answer for all of the following questions:

1. Interferons are a family of proteins that are
   A. not species specific.
   B. produced continuously.
   C. secreted in response to an inducer.
   D. targeted antiviral agents.

2. Alpha, beta, and gamma interferons differ in
   A. antigenic properties.
   B. ability to prevent viral infections.
   C. tumor specificity.
   D. cell of origin and method of generation.

3. Through altering the host's response to tumor cells, biological response modifiers
   A. effect nonspecific and specific immune responses.
   B. increase adverse side effects over time.
   C. change the basic behavior of tumor cells.
   D. predict response to treatment.

4. CD4 lymphocyte count is used primarily to
   A. determine when to initiate antiretroviral therapy.
   B. establish a prognosis.
   C. indicate presence of Kaposi's sarcoma.
   D. suggest risk factors for acquired immunodeficiency syndrome.

5. Colony stimulating factors given with chemotherapy may
   A. alleviate gastrointestinal side effects.
   B. permit moderate dose intensification of selected chemotherapeutic agents.
   C. prevent neutropenia.
   D. produce effects in pediatric and geriatric populations.

6. Which biological response modifier is only approved for use in clinical trials?
   A. Interferon-alpha.
   B. Granulocyte-macrophage colony stimulating factor (GM-CSF).
   C. Granulocyte colony stimulating factor (G-CSF).
   D. Tumor necrosis factor.

7. In a phase I clinical trial of a biological response modifier (BRM), which two broad effects are measured?
   A. Maximum tolerated dose and human response.
   B. Tumor response and nadir.
   C. Maximum tolerated dose and optimal immunomodulatory effect.
   D. Optimal immunomodulatory effect and nadir.

8. Most biological agents cause a flu-like syndrome that is characterized by the presence of the following symptoms:
   A. nausea/vomiting, diarrhea, myalgias.
   B. chills, fever, myalgias.
   C. headache, nausea/vomiting, diarrhea.
   D. fatigue, chills, anorexia.

9. Generally, the toxicities of biological response modifiers are directly related to
   A. dose, route, and duration.
   B. frequency, route, and duration.
   C. patient's prior history of concomitant illnesses.
   D. amount of tumor presence.

10. A major toxicity associated with high-dose interleukin-2 therapy is
   A. nausea/vomiting.
   B. decreased white blood cell count.
   C. capillary leak syndrome.
   D. increased red blood cell count.

1. *Answer:* **C**

   Rationale: Nucleated cells of vertebrates produce interferons when exposed to a virus. The virus is the inducer.

2. *Answer:* **D**

   Rationale: Alpha interferon is produced by B cells, T cells, macrophages, and null cells. Beta is produced by fibroblasts. Gamma is produced by T lymphocytes.

3. *Answer:* **A**

   Rationale: Biological response modifiers are a group of agents that modulate the immune system.

4. *Answer:* **A**

   Rationale: CD4 lymphocytes are helper cells. A decrease in the CD4 lymphocyte count indicates AIDS is developing.

5. *Answer:* **B**

   Rationale: Colony stimulating factors stimulate and regulate hematopoiesis. This function causes an increase in cell production which counterbalances cell kill from chemotherapeutic agents.

6. *Answer:* **D**

   Rationale: Interferon-alpha was FDA approved in 1987. GM-CSF and G-CSF were FDA approved in February, 1991. Tumor necrosis factor is still in clinical trials to determine therapeutic efficacy.

7. *Answer:* **C**

   Rationale: A phase I clinical trial with a BRM measures both the maximum tolerated dose and the optimal immunomodulatory effect of the agent.

8. *Answer:* **B**

   Rationale: The flu-like syndrome is characterized by chills, fever, and myalgias.

9. *Answer:* **A**

   Rationale: Toxicities associated with BRMs appear to be directly related to the dose, route, and duration of the agent administered.

10. *Answer:* **C**

    Rationale: High-dose interleukin-2 causes a decrease in systemic vascular resistance, producing a capillary leak syndrome with significant hypotension. Fluid replacement results in a significant weight gain with clinical presentation of peripheral edema, ascites, and possibly pulmonary interstial edema requiring intubation.

11. It is recommended that patients receiving GM-CSF or G-CSF have their CBC count monitored
    A. daily.
    B. every twelve hours.
    C. every other day.
    D. twice per week.

12. Which biological agent given in high doses can cause a diffuse pruritic desquamating rash?
    A. Interferon-alpha.
    B. Interleukin-2.
    C. Granulocyte-macrophage colony stimulating factor.
    D. Tumor necrosis factor.

13. Patients receiving G-CSF or GM-CSF may experience bone pain due to
    A. the rapid proliferation of white blood cells.
    B. the rapid proliferation of red blood cells.
    C. the rapid proliferation of platelets.
    D. all of the above.

14. Erythropoietin is contraindicated in patients who have
    A. reacted to red blood cell (RBC) transfusions.
    B. a history of uncontrolled hypertension.
    C. a history of anemia.
    D. active bleeding.

15. Which of the following cancers has shown the **BEST** therapeutic response to interleukin-2 therapy?
    A. Lymphoma.
    B. Renal cell cancer.
    C. Melanoma.
    D. Colon cancer.

Bone Marrow Transplantation

Kathy E. Coyle

Select the BEST answer for all of the following questions:

1. Granulocyte-macrophage colony stimulating factor (GM-CSF) is a biological response modifier that is being used in autologous transplant patients. This drug stimulates the growth of
    A. erythrocytes.
    B. platelets.
    C. neutrophils.
    D. lymphocytes.

2. The most desirable source of donor marrow to treat acute lymphocytic leukemia is
    A. syngeneic.
    B. autologous.
    C. allogeneic.
    D. cadaveric.

3. GM-CSF is used for all of the following reasons **EXCEPT**
    A. hospital stays may be shortened.
    B. patients may be at decreased risk for infections.
    C. less blood products will be administered.
    D. graft failure may be reversed.

4. Autologous marrow transplantations are now being performed on all of the following diseases **EXCEPT**
    A. aplastic anemia.
    B. neuroblastoma.
    C. lymphoma.
    D. leukemia.

11. *Answer:* **D**

Rationale: Amgen, Immunex, and Hoechst-Roussel all recommend twice weekly monitoring of CBC counts in order to avoid excessive leukocytosis.

12. *Answer:* **B**

Rationale: Interleukin-2 administered at high doses causes the development of diffuse erythema that evolves into a pruritic desquamating rash.

13. *Answer:* **A**

Rationale: G-CSF and GM-CSF produce a rapid proliferation of white blood cells in the marrow, resulting in bone pain.

14. *Answer:* **B**

Rationale: Erythropoietin is contraindicated in patients with a history of uncontrolled hypertension because blood pressure may increase during the initiation of treatment when the hematocrit is rising.

15. *Answer:* **B**

Rationale: Clinical trials have reported a 30% response rate for renal cell carcinoma treated with interleukin-2. This is a higher rate than that reported for the other cancers listed.

REFERENCES

Abernathy E, (1987). Biotherapy: An Introductory Overview. *Oncology Nursing Forum.* 14 (6): S13–15.

——, (1989). *Biological Response Modifier Guidelines and Recommendations for Nursing Education and Practice.* Pittsburgh: Oncology Nursing Society.

Brophy L, Rieger PT, (1992). Implications of Biological Response Modifier Therapy for Nursing, in, Clark JC, McGee RF, (eds). *Core Curriculum for Oncology Nursing,* (2nd ed). Philadelphia: WB Saunders.

Bucholtz J, (1987). Radiolabeled Antibody Therapy. *Seminars in Oncology Nursing.* 3 (1): 67–73.

Dewey D, (1987). Role of the Nurse in the Use of Biological Response Modifiers. *American Association of Occupational Health Nurses Journal.* 35 (4): 163–167.

Dillman JB, (1988). Toxicity of Monoclonal Antibodies in the Treatment of Cancer. *Seminars in Oncology Nursing.* 12 (2): 107–111.

Dillman JB, (1989). New Antineoplastic Therapies and Inherent Risks: Monoclonal Antibodies, Biologic Response Modifiers and Interleukin-2. *Journal of Intravenous Nursing.* 12 (2): 103–113.

Hahn MB, Jassak PF, (1988). Nursing Management of Patients Receiving Interferon. *Seminars in Oncology Nursing.* 4 (2): 95–101.

Haeuber D, DiJulio JE, (1989). Hematopoietic Colony Stimulating Factors: An Overview. *Oncology Nursing Forum.* 16 (2): 247–255.

Haeuber D, (1989). Recent Advances in the Management of Biotherapy-related Side-effects: Flu-like Syndrome. *Oncology Nursing Forum.* 16 (6): S35–41.

Hood LE, Abernathy E, (1991). Biologic Response Modifiers, in, Baird SB, McCorkle R, Grant M, (eds). *Cancer Nursing: A Comprehensive Textbook.* Philadephia: WB Saunders, pp. 321–343.

Irwin MM, (1987). Patients Receiving Biological Response Modifiers: Overview of Nursing Care. *Oncology Nursing Forum.* 14 (6): S32–37.

Jassak PF, Sticklin LA, (1987). Interleukin-2: An Overview. *Oncology Nursing Forum.* 13 (6): 17–22.

Jassak PF, (1991). Knowledge Deficit Related to Biotherapy, in, McNally JC, Somerville ET, Miaskowski C, Rostad M, (eds). *Guidelines for Oncology Nursing Practice,* (2nd ed). Philadelphia: WB Saunders, pp. 76–79.

Moldawer NP, Figlin RA, (1988). Tumor Necrosis Factor: Current Clinical Status and Implications for Nursing Management. *Seminars in Oncology Nursing.* 4 (2): 120–125.

Bone Marrow Transplantation

1. *Answer:* **C**

Rationale: Neutrophils are a part of the granulocyte line of cells that can be stimulated by GM-CSF.

2. *Answer:* **A**

Rationale: A syngeneic transplant decreases the patient's risk of developing graft-versus-host-disease and relapse.

3. *Answer:* **C**

Rationale: GM-CSF does not directly affect the production of red blood cells or platelets and, as such, does not decrease the need for blood components.

4. *Answer:* **A**

Rationale: Autologous marrow transplant requires an adequate harvest of marrow stem cells. These cells are lacking in patients diagnosed with aplastic anemia.

5. The organism most commonly responsible for interstitial pneumonia in the bone marrow transplant patient is a
   A. bacteria.
   B. fungus.
   C. virus.
   D. protozoan.

6. Your patient is being treated with cyclophosphamide as part of the preparative regimen for bone marrow transplantation. She is becoming confused and lethargic; her weight has increased from yesterday but no edema is present; you note her sodium has fallen from 140 to 129; you might suspect
   A. graft-versus-host-disease (GVHD).
   B. severe combined immune deficiency syndrome.
   C. hemorrhagic cystitis.
   D. syndrome of inappropriate antidiuretic hormone (SIADH).

7. Neutropenia, post-transplant immunosuppression, and disruption of mucosal barriers, all combined, increase the bone marrow transplant patient's risk for
   A. graft versus host disease.
   B. veno-occlusive disease.
   C. relapse.
   D. infections.

8. Your patient received a central line ten days ago and an allogeneic bone marrow transplant seven days ago. When changing the central line dressing, you note the exit site is red, raised, and, on palpation, a serosanguinous drainage appears but no pus. The patient's last temperature was 38.3°C. You determine that these signs are
   A. normal and the tunnel probably is healing.
   B. abnormal and the site should be cultured for possible infection.
   C. normal and probably due to catheter manipulation.
   D. abnormal and can indicate an allergic reaction to the catheter.

9. The purpose of using high-dose chemotherapy and/or radiation therapy in bone marrow transplantation includes all of the following **EXCEPT**
   A. making space in the bone marrow.
   B. immunosuppression of the patient.
   C. destroying any residual tumor cells.
   D. preventing veno-occlusive disease.

10. Acute graft-versus-host-disease primarily affects which organ systems?
   A. Skin, lungs, and GI tract.
   B. Liver, lungs, and GI tract.
   C. Skin, liver, and lungs.
   D. Skin, liver, and GI tract.

11. Which cells are thought to be responsible for graft-versus-host-disease?
   A. B cells.
   B. Granulocytes.
   C. T cells.
   D. Macrophages.

12. Which of the following are symptoms of veno-occlusive disease (VOD)?
   A. Sudden weight gain, ascites, and jaundice.
   B. Encephalopathy, interstitial pneumonitis, and ascites.
   C. Right upper quadrant pain, jaundice, and maculopapular rash.
   D. Sudden weight gain, pulmonary edema, and encephalopathy.

13. Total body irradiation (TBI) can cause all of the following side effects **EXCEPT**
   A. SIADH.
   B. altered growth and development.
   C. sterility.
   D. cataracts.

14. If a patient receives an allogeneic transplant from an HLA-identical donor but the donor has a different ABO blood type,
   A. the patient will reject the marrow.
   B. the patient will convert to the donor's blood type.
   C. the patient will have GVHD and ABO-incompatible marrow.
   D. the donor's blood type will change to the patient's.

5. *Answer:* **C**

Rationale: While all of the organisms listed can produce interstitial pneumonia, viruses are the most frequently *documented* cause of interstitial pneumonia.

6. *Answer:* **D**

Rationale: Excess free water leads to a dilute hyponatremic serum. This excess is intracellular, leading to cellular swelling, particularly within the CNS, resulting in confusion and disorientation. Weight gain, without edema, results from the fluid shift to the intracellular spaces.

7. *Answer:* **D**

Rationale: Neutropenia, immunosuppression, and mucosal barrier disruption increase the potential for infection because of altered protective mechanisms.

8. *Answer:* **B**

Rationale: The patient is most likely still severely neutropenic and unable to produce pus indicative of infection. The line should be cultured for possible infection.

9. *Answer:* **D**

Rationale: Veno-occlusive disease is a complication of high-dose chemotherapy administration. The other responses are the goals of the preparatory regimen for bone marrow transplantation.

10. *Answer:* **D**

Rationale: Acute GVHD primarily affects the skin, gut, and liver. The lungs may sometimes be affected by chronic GVHD.

11. *Answer:* **C**

Rationale: It appears that T cells release endogenous interferons that provide the stimulus for the expression of MHC antigens. This promotes recognition of the host as foreign, resulting in GVHD.

12. *Answer:* **A**

Rationale: Sudden weight gain, ascites, and jaundice are hallmarks of VOD, which is not associated with pneumonitis, pulmonary edema, or a maculopapular rash.

13. *Answer:* **A**

Rationale: Responses B, C, and D are side effects directly related to total body irradiation (TBI). TBI has no effect on the development of SIADH.

14. *Answer:* **B**

Rationale: As the donor's immune and ABO systems begin to engraft, the donor's ABO will replace the patient's.

15. Which of the following is **NOT** a primary symptom of chronic graft-versus-host-disease?
   A. Damaged lacrimal glands.
   B. Scleroderma-like skin condition.
   C. Leukemic relapse.
   D. Chronic liver failure.

16. Your patient is day +17 post an allogeneic transplant. You note a fine maculopapular rash over the palms and soles. The stool output is increased and watery. The WBC is 400. The patient has been on vancomycin for five days. You suspect
   A. drug reaction.
   B. septic eruptions.
   C. hypersensitivity reaction.
   D. acute graft-versus-host-disease.

17. Which drug is not used to prevent graft-versus-host-disease?
   A. Methotrexate.
   B. Cyclosporin A.
   C. Cyclophosphamide.
   D. Prednisone.

18. Which of the following is usually **NOT** a complication of an autologous bone marrow transplant?
   A. Delayed engraftment.
   B. Graft-versus-host-disease.
   C. Infection.
   D. Marrow aplasia.

19. Which of the following is a **TRUE** statement about autologous bone marrow transplant?
   A. Autologous transplantation is sometimes called a "bone marrow rescue."
   B. Preparation for autologous bone marrow transplant never includes total body irradiation.
   C. Marrow for the procedure is collected only when the patient is in remission.
   D. Marrow is donated by a sibling.

20. The purpose of "treating" or "purging" autologous bone marrow is to prevent
   A. graft-versus-host-disease.
   B. reinfusion of malignant cells.
   C. graft rejection.
   D. veno-occlusive disease.

21. Allogeneic bone marrow transplant recipients who develop acute graft-versus-host-disease have a lower relapse rate. This is probably due to
   A. cyclosporin administration.
   B. graft versus leukemia effect.
   C. high-dose steroids.
   D. methotrexate.

22. Allogeneic bone marrow transplants (BMT) differ from all other forms of BMT because
   A. the host can recognize the graft and reject it.
   B. the graft can recognize the host and reject it.
   C. due to HLA typing, no rejection occurs.
   D. the patient's own marrow is used and no rejection occurs.

23. Which of the following measures has **NOT** been successful in preventing cytomegalovirus (CMV) infection in bone marrow transplantation patients?
   A. Giving the patient total body irradiation in fractionated doses.
   B. Giving the patient immunoglobulin before and after the marrow transplant.
   C. Giving the patient antiviral drugs.
   D. Giving the patient only CMV seronegative blood products.

24. All of the following are "purging" agents for autologous bone marrow **EXCEPT**
   A. monoclonal antibodies.
   B. 4-hydroperoxycyclophamide.
   C. sheep red blood cells.
   D. magnetic beads.

15. *Answer:* **C**

Rationale: Scleroderma itself is not a primary symptom of GVHD, but a scleroderma-like condition does result. Leukemic relapse is not a symptom of chronic GVHD.

16. *Answer:* **D**

Rationale: Acute GVHD may occur anytime around day +14 and is characterized by a rash on palms and soles as well as increased, watery diarrhea.

17. *Answer:* **C**

Rationale: Cyclophosphamide is used in pretransplant conditioning regimens. All other drugs are used in prevention of GVHD.

18. *Answer:* **B**

Rationale: Autologous marrow does not generally recognize the host as foreign, the typical situation resulting in GVHD.

19. *Answer:* **A**

Rationale: Responses B, C, and D are not valid statements about autologous bone marrow transplant.

20. *Answer:* **B**

Rationale: The reason for purging autologous bone marrow is to remove malignant cells. If all the malignant cells are not destroyed, malignant cells may be reinfused, which leads to relapse.

21. *Answer:* **B**

Rationale: Patients who develop GVHD, in the acute form, have been reported to have had leukemic cells disappear.

22. *Answer:* **B**

Rationale: The immunocompetent T lymphocytes in the graft (donor) recognize the immunocompetent tissues of the host (patient) as foreign and mount an immunological reaction against the host.

23. *Answer:* **A**

Rationale: Responses B, C, and D all are methods used to prevent CMV; response A does not play a role.

24. *Answer:* **C**

Rationale: All responses except C are methods for removing malignant cells from marrow harvests.

REFERENCES

Buchsel PC, Kelleher J, (1989). Bone Marrow Transplantation. *Nursing Clinics of North America.* 24 (4): 907–937.

Davis BV, (1991). Injury, Potential for, Related to Graft Versus Host Disease (GVHD), in, McNally JC, Somerville ET, Miaskowski C, Rostad M, (eds). *Guidelines for Cancer Nursing Practice,* (2nd ed). Philadelphia: WB Saunders, pp. 223–230.

Ford R, Ballard B, (1988). Acute Complications after Bone Marrow Transplantation. *Seminars in Oncology Nursing.* 4 (1): 15–24.

Ford R, Eissenberg S, (1990). Bone Marrow Transplant Recent Advances and Nursing Implications. *Nursing Clinics of North America.* 25 (2): 405–422.

Ford RC, (1991). Bone Marrow Transplantation, in, Baird SB, McCorkle R, Grant M, (eds). *Cancer Nursing: A Comprehensive Textbook.* Philadephia: WB Saunders, pp. 385–406.

Gurevich I, Tafuro P, (1986). The Comprised Host Deficit Specific Infection and the Spectrum of Prevention. *Cancer Nursing.* 9 (5): 263–275.

Somerville ET (1991). Knowledge Deficit Related to Bone Marrow Transplant, in, McNally JC, Somerville ET, Miaskowski C, Rostad M, (eds). *Guidelines for Oncology Nursing Practice,* (2nd ed). Philadelphia: WB Saunders, pp. 85–94.

Wilkie T, Coyle K, Shapiro D, (1990). Bone Marrow Transplantation Today and Tomorrow. *American Journal of Nursing.* 90 (5): 48–58.

Wikle T, (1992). Implications of Bone Marrow Transplantation for Nursing, in, Clark JC, McGee RF, (eds). *Core Curriculum for Oncology Nursing,* (2nd ed). Philadelphia: WB Saunders.

Unproven Methods

Nancy E. Kane

Select the BEST answer for all of the following questions:

1. Mr. S, diagnosed with testicular cancer, completed chemotherapy and radiation last year and has recently been diagnosed with a recurrence in his lungs. Since his initial treatment, he has used relaxation and imagery, along with a macrobiotic diet, to "help keep the cancer from coming back." He now states, "There's no point in going through more chemo. I'm going to stick to the diet and imagery. That's as good as anything." The best response to give Mr. S would be:
   A. "I can't understand why you want to use that since it didn't work before."
   B. "I can understand how you feel since you've failed chemo anyway."
   C. "I can understand how you feel right now. Tell me more about why you feel this way."
   D. "I guess it really doesn't matter what you do at this point."

2. Strategies that may be employed to reduce the risk of clients seeking unproven methods include all of the following **EXCEPT** to
   A. provide literature on unproven methods to clients and families.
   B. establish cancer support and education programs and groups in the community.
   C. limit discussion of unproven methods to help discourage their use.
   D. foster open communication between the client and family and the health care team.

3. Clients who may be at risk for using unproven methods of cancer treatment include
   A. clients who have had a difficult time tolerating the side effects of previous treatment.
   B. clients who are uninformed about their disease and treatment.
   C. clients with advanced disease for which cure is not possible.
   D. all of the above.

4. What percentage of the U.S. population is estimated to seek unproven cancer treatment?
   A. 10%.
   B. 25%.
   C. 50%.
   D. 75%.

5. Mrs. G has advanced breast cancer and returns to the office for a visit. She brings with her an article from a "women's magazine" regarding a dietary treatment for cancer. She asks whether or not to follow the treatment. Which of the following is the best advice to give Mrs. G?
   A. "You shouldn't believe what you read in that kind of magazine related to cancer treatment."
   B. "I've never heard of that treatment and would not advise you to follow it."
   C. "Let's look at it together and see what it says."
   D. "Why not try it. It certainly can't hurt."

1. *Answer:* **C**

    Rationale: A high-risk time for patients is when the goals of treatment shift from cure to palliation. Mr. S is aware that his chance of cure is much different now, and he feels hopeless. Responses A, B, and D accentuate that hopeless feeling as well as potentially inducing guilt about depending on alternative methods in the past. Response C encourages Mr. S to discuss his feelings and increases the chance of maintaining a supportive relationship with him.

2. *Answer:* **C**

    Rationale: Although the impulse is to avoid discussion of unproven methods for fear of validating their use, initiating such discussions often demystifies the treatment and provides a time for teaching and support. Providing literature also allows and encourages discussion. Including the topic in support/education programs provides a forum for education and mutual support.

3. *Answer:* **D**

    Rationale: There are no stereotypes for those who seek unproven methods. All patients should be viewed as "at risk."

4. *Answer:* **C**

    Rationale: This question defines the scope of the problem and underscores that there are no stereotypes for seekers of unproven treatments.

5. *Answer:* **C**

    Rationale: When a client asks for advice about unproven treatment, it is an opportunity for assessment, education, and support. Responses A and B effectively close the door to any future discussion on this topic. Since unproven methods of any type may not be innocuous and may have detrimental physical effects, response D should not be offered without careful evaluation.

6. Mr. J is newly diagnosed with non-Hodgkin's lymphoma. He and his wife have changed their usual diet and are following a diet prescribed by a nutritionist in the community. Mr. J is also taking supplemental megavitamins prescribed by the same person. He and his wife are questioning whether to continue with the radiation and chemotherapy, or to abandon it and rely only on diet and vitamins. They ask for advice. The best advice to give them would be:

    A. "Diet and vitamin treatment will not help your cancer, and I think you should stop it."

    B. "The radiation and chemotherapy you are taking is based on scientific principles; the diet/vitamin treatment is not."

    C. "It's important that you continue the chemotherapy and radiation. Why not stop the diet and vitamins and see how you feel."

    D. "I'm glad you talked to me about this. Let's talk about all of these treatments and figure out the best plan to follow."

7. A nurse is speaking to a group of factory employees on behalf of the American Cancer Society. Someone in the audience asks, "Why are you doctors and nurses so down on things like laetrile and vitamins? You have no cure for cancer, so why not let people use whatever they want?" The best response would be:

    A. "You're right. We have no cure for cancer, but that doesn't justify the use of such treatments."

    B. "That's a good point. Let's talk about some of the pros and cons of unproven treatments."

    C. "I hear what you're saying, but those treatments aren't based on any scientific fact."

    D. "That's a good point. With some cancers, it really doesn't matter what the person uses."

8. Examples of unproven methods of cancer treatment include all of the following **EXCEPT**

    A. immuno-augmentation therapy (IAT).
    B. levamisole.
    C. laetrile.
    D. macrobiotic diet.

Supportive Therapies and Procedures

Lynn Erdman, Marcia E. Rostad, and Leslie B. Tyson

Select the BEST answer for all of the following questions:

1. Mr. J is receiving his second unit of packed red blood cells for Hgb/Hct of 8/24. He is complaining of itching. His temperature is 100°F orally. Which is the most appropriate action to take **FIRST**?

    A. Stop the infusion of packed red blood cells.
    B. Administer acetaminophen and diphenhydramine hydrochloride.
    C. Notify the physician.
    D. Open another IV line with 0.9% saline.

2. Your patient has disseminated intravascular coagulation (DIC) with a platelet count of 10,000, Hgb of 7, PTT of 40, and is actively bleeding. You should be prepared to give all of the following blood products **EXCEPT**

    A. packed red blood cells.
    B. platelets.
    C. fresh frozen plasma.
    D. white blood cells.

6.   *Answer:* **D**

Rationale: This vignette illustrates several points. First, there is no stereotype of a seeker of unproven treatment. Second, if clients do seek them, we must find out why they do. Third, there is literature to support that when people feel more control over their situation, they will be less inclined toward abandoning "traditional" therapy for unproven treatment.

7.   *Answer:* **B**

Rationale: Many people believe the health care establishment is not moving fast enough to "cure cancer" or to provide less toxic treatments. They may not be concerned about the scientific underpinnings or understand them. Also, cancer is still viewed by much of the public as a uniformly fatal disease in which treatment ultimately makes no difference. Using such a forum to educate the public, and not to discourage such inquiry, is an important component of the nurse's role in public education.

8.   *Answer:* **B**

Rationale: Responses A, B, and D are common unproven methods. Levamisole is indicated in the treatment of colon cancer with 5FU.

REFERENCES

Bridgen ML, (1987). Unorthodox Therapy and Your Cancer Patient. *Postgraduate Medicine*. 81 (1): 271–280.

Cassileth BR, (1989). The Social Implications of Questionable Cancer Therapies. *Cancer*. 63 (7): 1247–1250.

Cassileth BR, Brown H, (1988). Unorthodox Cancer Medicine. *CA*. 38 (3): 176–186.

Cassileth BR, Kleenbart JM, (1991). Questionable Cancer Therapies, in, Baird SB, McCorkle R, Grant M, (eds). *Cancer Nursing: A Comprehensive Textbook*. Philadephia: WB Saunders, pp. 415–424.

Danielson KJ, Stewart DE, Lippert GP, (1988). Unconventional Cancer Remedies. *Canadian Medical Association Journal*. 138 (1): 1005–1011.

Hiratzka S, (1985). Knowledge and Attitudes of Persons with Cancer Towards Use of Unproven Treatment Methods. *Oncology Nursing Forum*. 12 (1): 36–41.

Howard-Ruben J, Miller N, (1984). Unproven Methods of Cancer Management. Part II: Current Trends and Implications for Patient Care. *Oncology Nursing Forum*. 11 (1): 67–74.

Kane N, (1992). Implications of Unproven Methods for Nursing, in, Clark JC, McGee RF, (eds). *Core Curriculum for Oncology Nursing*, (2nd ed). Philadelphia: WB Saunders.

Miller N, Howard-Rubin J, (1984). Unproven Methods of Cancer Management. Part I: Background and Historical Perspective. *Oncology Nursing Forum*. 10 (4): 46–54.

Wajtalewicz-Friedberg K, Flynn BA, Riley MB, Kelley CM, Roth EL, (1991). Knowledge Deficit Related to Unproven Methods of Cancer Treatment, in, McNally JC, Somerville ET, Miaskowski C, Rostad M, (eds). *Guidelines for Oncology Nursing Practice*, (2nd ed). Philadelphia: WB Saunders, pp. 97–100.

Supportive Therapies and Procedures

1.   *Answer:* **A**

Rationale: All may be appropriate actions, however, *first* is the key word in this question. The first action should be to stop the infusion and evaluate the symptoms in order to prevent a more serious reaction from occurring.

2.   *Answer:* **D**

Rationale: White blood cells would not be indicated in the clinical situation described.

3.   Mr. S has leukemia and has had numerous blood transfusions with multiple febrile reactions. He is to receive four units of packed red blood cells. His temperature is 97.6°F, pulse = 88, and respirations = 20. He should receive the blood through
   A.   a leukocyte depletion filter.
   B.   straight IV tubing.
   C.   a pressure pump.
   D.   a blood warmer.

4.   Mr. L is admitted with a platelet count of 8000 and a nosebleed. Random donor platelets indicate that Mr. L should
   A.   increase his platelet count.
   B.   decrease his risk of alloimmunization.
   C.   increase his hemoglobin.
   D.   decrease his risk of infection.

5.   All of the following are symptoms indicating the need for a blood transfusion **EXCEPT**
   A.   bruising.
   B.   fatigue.
   C.   decreased pulse and increased blood pressure.
   D.   bleeding.

6.   Signs of cachexia include all of the following **EXCEPT**
   A.   weight loss greater than 10% of ideal body weight.
   B.   tissue wasting.
   C.   anorexia.
   D.   nausea and vomiting.

7.   A common controversy about nutritional support for the cancer patient is that nutritional support
   A.   feeds the tumor, encouraging growth.
   B.   is a long-term benefit.
   C.   predisposes the patient to infection.
   D.   is all of the above.

8.   A potential side effect of abruptly stopping total parenteral nutrition (TPN) is
   A.   hyperglycemia.
   B.   hypoglycemia.
   C.   shaking chills.
   D.   diarrhea.

9.   TPN is commonly used in the patient with cancer for all of the following reasons **EXCEPT**
   A.   pre/post-operative support.
   B.   loss of GI function.
   C.   weight loss greater than 10% of ideal body weight.
   D.   supplementation of oral intake.

10.   The **MOST** common side effect of administering enteral feedings too rapidly is
   A.   constipation.
   B.   vomiting.
   C.   diarrhea.
   D.   alopecia.

11.   Which statement is **TRUE** regarding TPN at home?
   A.   Vascular access devices used for TPN have higher infection rates.
   B.   People on TPN tend to have longer survival rates than those who do not receive TPN.
   C.   Home TPN is generally not reimbursable by most third-party payors.
   D.   TPN has not been shown to prolong survival or impact on tumor response.

12.   A **COMMON** side effect of amphotericin B given through a central line is
   A.   shaking chills.
   B.   vomiting.
   C.   phlebitis.
   D.   hypoglycemia.

13.   Mrs. J has breast cancer and is being treated with chemotherapy. Her WBC ten days after her last treatment is 800. Her physician prescribes prophylactic antibiotics to be given at home. Which is an appropriate statement for you to teach Mrs. J?
   A.   Discontinue daily temperature monitoring during antibiotic therapy.
   B.   Take all of her daily antibiotic doses between 8 AM and 5 PM.
   C.   Notify the physician of any rash, fever, or nausea that she may experience.
   D.   Chills are an expected side effect of antibiotic therapy.

3. *Answer:* **A**

   Rationale: Use of a leukocyte depletion filter removes the white blood cells from blood and decreases the chance of transfusion reaction.

4. *Answer:* **A**

   Rationale: Random donor platelets do not decrease the risk of alloimmunization. Single donor platelets provide less exposure to foreign antigens, hence decreasing the risk for the development of alloimmunization.

5. *Answer:* **C**

   Rationale: As the Hgb drops, the circulation of blood diminishes and, therefore, the cardiac output begins to increase in patients with an Hgb below 10. Thus, patients experience an increased pulse and decreased blood pressure.

6. *Answer:* **D**

   Rationale: The key is *signs* of cachexia. The other answers may be symptoms of cachexia, but they are not warning signs.

7. *Answer:* **D**

   Rationale: Controversies involve all of the areas identified.

8. *Answer:* **B**

   Rationale: Insulin production increases with TPN, and it will halt abruptly if TPN is stopped quickly. With too much insulin on board, the body will react by going into hypoglycemia.

9. *Answer:* **D**

   Rationale: If the GI tract is functioning, another route of administration for supplemental feeding should be used.

10. *Answer:* **C**

    Rationale: Rapid infusion of enteral feedings overstimulates the GI function, and the result is the rapid excretion of the feeding, resulting in diarrhea.

11. *Answer:* **D**

    Rationale: Studies have not shown an increase in survival rate or a decrease in tumor size due to TPN administration.

12. *Answer:* **A**

    Rationale: Phlebitis is not a problem when amphotericin B is given through a central line. Responses B and D are not side effects of amphotericin B.

13. *Answer:* **C**

    Rationale: Rash, fever, and nausea may indicate a reaction to the antibiotic or may indicate another infectious process. The physician would need to be aware of these symptoms in order to treat the patient appropriately.

14. Vancomycin can cause all of these effects **EXCEPT**:
    A. anaphylaxis.
    B. extravasation.
    C. rash.
    D. nausea.

15. Amphotericin B and fluconazole are two common agents used for the treatment of
    A. staphylococcus.
    B. candida albicans.
    C. streptococcus.
    D. *E. coli.*

16. Mrs. L received her fourth chemotherapy treatment for ovarian cancer two weeks ago. Her absolute granulocyte count is 800, and she calls the office complaining of a temperature of 38°C. What would you advise her to do?
    A. Drink 8 oz of clear fluids every two hours while awake.
    B. Take two 350-mg acetaminophen tabs.
    C. Take a cool, tepid bath and two 350-mg acetaminophen tabs.
    D. Come in to the office and see the physician immediately.

17. Gentamycin and tobramycin are used in the treatment of Pseudomonas infections in patients with cancer. The major toxicity of these agents is
    A. ototoxicity.
    B. cardiac toxicity.
    C. nephrotoxicity.
    D. neurotoxicity.

18. Strict isolation is appropriate protection in which situation?
    A. Neutropenia.
    B. Varicella.
    C. Tuberculosis.
    D. Hepatitis B.

19. A 44-year-old woman with ovarian cancer has a temporary epidural catheter for pain control. She has agreed to have a long-term device placed to maintain her epidural analgesia. All of the following devices are appropriate for long-term epidural pain management **EXCEPT**
    A. implanted port.
    B. tunneled epidural catheter.
    C. PCA pump.
    D. implanted infusion pump.

20. One hour after putting urokinase into an occluded central venous catheter, the catheter remains occluded when the nurse attempts to withdraw the urokinase. The nurse should
    A. try to force the catheter open with a normal saline flush.
    B. send the patient home with instructions to increase the frequency of heparin flushes.
    C. refer the patient for insertion of a new catheter.
    D. obtain a physician's order for a second dose of urokinase.

21. A change in the rate of infusion of an implanted infusion pump can be attributed to:
    A. a change in elevation and prolonged fever.
    B. a change in arterial pressure and a change in volume.
    C. a change in volume and prolonged fever.
    D. a change in arterial pressure and prolonged fever.

22. Which of the following clinical uses is **NOT** an appropriate indication for placement of a long-term catheter?
    A. Continuous infusions of vesicant chemotherapy.
    B. Infrequent administration of intravenous therapy and medications.
    C. Intensive outpatient intravenous therapies.
    D. Frequent and intensive intravenous therapy.

14. *Answer:* **B**

Rationale: Extravasation is not a side effect of vancomycin administration.

15. *Answer:* **B**

Rationale: These are antifungal agents and candida is a fungal organism.

16. *Answer:* **D**

Rationale: Immediate treatment must be initiated for the neutropenic patient with a fever.

17. *Answer:* **C**

Rationale: The major problem with the use of gentamycin and tobramycin is nephrotoxicity. Careful monitoring of antibiotic levels and urine output is indicated to maximize treatment while minimizing toxicity.

18. *Answer:* **B**

Rationale: Isolation techniques must be appropriate for the causative infectious organism. Tuberculosis requires respiratory isolation and hepatitis B requires the use of universal precautions, whereas neutropenia mandates protective isolation.

19. *Answer:* **C**

Rationale: The PCA pump delivers the medication but does not provide access to the epidural space.

20. *Answer:* **D**

Rationale: If urokinase is not successful after one hour, it is recommended that a second dose of urokinase be administered.

21. *Answer:* **D**

Rationale: Response D identifies the factors that can cause a change in the infusion rate of an implanted infusion pump.

22. *Answer:* **B**

Rationale: Permanent, long-term catheters are not indicated for infrequent use, due to the cost of placement and maintenance and potential risks involved.

23.   Mr. C is receiving total parenteral nutrition (TPN) infusion via a large-volume infusion system into an implanted port. During the infusion, an alarm sounds from the infusion pump. On inspection, you note that the pump is signaling an occlusion. Which of the following is **NOT** a likely cause of the alarm?

A.   An occlusion has occurred in the infusion system tubing.

B.   The needle into the port has become partially dislodged.

C.   The implanted port catheter has become occluded.

D.   The infusion system is inappropriate for infusing TPN.

24.   A patient discharged on intermittent intravenous infusions of ceftazidime would best be managed by a

A.   small-volume infusion system.

B.   large-volume infusion system.

C.   patient-controlled infusion system.

D.   variable-rate infusion system.

25.   A patient is receiving subcutaneous infusions of morphine. This patient should be regularly assessed for signs and symptoms of subcutaneous tissue irritation, including all of the following **EXCEPT**

A.   local temperature change.

B.   rash.

C.   edema.

D.   burning.

26.   A patient connected to a patient-controlled analgesia pump (PCA) suddenly complains of an increase in pain. Possible causes include all of the following **EXCEPT**

A.   mechanical failure of the pump.

B.   disconnected tubing.

C.   inappropriate program setting.

D.   tolerance to the drug.

27.   Twenty-four hours post-placement of an implanted port, the patient presents with regional discomfort, pain, and swelling at the site of the port. The patient's vital signs are within normal limits except for a temperature of 37.2°C. Likely problems include all of the following **EXCEPT**

A.   pocket infection.

B.   port–catheter separation.

C.   venous thrombosis.

D.   trauma to the site.

28.   A leukemia patient, who recently received high-dose cytarabine, presents with a fever and a slightly reddened central venous catheter site. You suspect the fever is **PRIMARILY** due to

A.   a possible central venous catheter site infection secondary to chemotherapy-induced neutropenia.

B.   a possible central venous catheter infection secondary to poor catheter exit site care.

C.   a common side effect of cytarabine.

D.   a fast-growing malignancy unresponsive to chemotherapy.

29.   A patient who recently received chemotherapy presents with a 38°C temperature and a white blood cell count of 2500 with 10% segs and 8% bands. The nurse concludes that

A.   the patient has an infection secondary to neutropenia.

B.   the tumor is aggressively growing, raising the body temperature and suppressing the immune system.

C.   the patient has a gram-negative infection.

D.   the fever should resolve because of an adequate leukocyte count.

23. *Answer:* **D**

Rationale: When an occlusion alarm occurs on a patient receiving infusions through a port, responses A, B, and C are likely causes that should be investigated.

24. *Answer:* **A**

Rationale: Since ceftazidime is an antibiotic administered at 8 to 12 hr intervals, a small-volume infusion system would meet the patient's needs.

25. *Answer:* **D**

Rationale: Burning is not a symptom of subcutaneous tissue irritation caused by morphine.

26. *Answer:* **D**

Rationale: PCA pumps are not indicated for use in chronic pain where patients are most likely to develop drug tolerance. Responses A, B, and C reflect pump malfunctions that may prevent delivery of the programmed dose of morphine.

27. *Answer:* **B**

Rationale: Responses A, C, and D could explain the symptoms experienced. A temperature would not be indicative of a port–catheter separation.

28. *Answer:* **A**

Rationale: Catheter exit site infection frequently occurs during the neutropenic phase after chemotherapy.

29. *Answer:* **A**

Rationale: The patient's absolute neutrophil count is 450, and he is at high risk for infection, indicated by a temperature of 38°C.

30. Mrs. L was hospitalized for the insertion of a central venous catheter and the administration of nitrogen mustard and vincristine. Ten days after discharge, Mrs. L telephones crying that the catheter site is red and painful. She adds, "I took good care of the catheter. What did I do wrong?" Which of the following is the **BEST** response to her statements?

    A. "You may have picked up an infection while hospitalized."

    B. "You probably forgot to wash your hands before caring for your catheter."

    C. "The chemotherapy has lowered your blood cell count, which made you susceptible to an infection."

    D. "Infections after surgery commonly occur in patients with cancer."

31. The source of the contaminate in an endogenous infection is

    A. the host.

    B. another person.

    C. hospital equipment.

    D. insects or animals.

32. The nurse is protected from contact with infectious materials by

    A. placing all oncology patients in strict isolation.

    B. drawing daily CBC on oncology patients to determine the level of neutropenia.

    C. practicing universal precautions.

    D. using only disposable equipment.

30. *Answer:* **C**

Rationale: The oncology nurse troubleshoots problems related to the catheter and provides reassurance to patients, avoiding statements that imply guilt or blame.

31. *Answer:* **A**

Rationale: Oncology patients become immunosuppressed secondary to chemotherapy or radiotherapy, making them susceptible to infection originating from organisms normally present in the body.

32. *Answer:* **C**

Rationale: Universal precautions are the minimal standard of protection required for all health care providers.

REFERENCES

Adams F, et al., (1989). Focal Subdermal Toxicity with Subcutaneous Opiod Infusion in Patients with Cancer Pain. *Journal of Pain and Symptom Management.* 3: 31–33.

Alexander EJ, (1991). Injury, Potential for, Related to Thrombocytopenia, in, McNally JC, Somerville ET, Miaskowski C, Rostad M, (eds). *Guidelines for Oncology Nursing Practice,* (2nd ed). Philadelphia: WB Saunders, pp. 203–207.

Bodey GP, (1989). Evolution of Antibiotic Therapy for Infection in Neutropenic Patients: Studies at MD Anderson Hospital. *Review of Infectious Diseases.* 11 (7): S1582–S1590.

Burt M, Gorschboth C, (1982). A Controlled Prospective Randomized Trial Evaluating the Metabolic Effects of Enteral and Parenteral Nutrition in the Cancer Patient. *Cancer.* 49 (6): 1092–1105.

Deiseroth A, Walterstein Jr. R, (1989). Use of Blood and Blood Products, in, DeVita VT, Hellman S, Rosenberg S, (eds). *Cancer Principles and Practice,* (3rd ed). Philadelphia: JB Lippincott, pp. 2045–2055.

Donovan CT, (1982). Protective Isolation. *Oncology Nursing Forum.* 9 (3): 50–53.

Ellerhorst-Ryan JM, (1985). Complications of the Myeloproliferative System: Infection and Sepsis. *Seminars in Oncology Nursing.* 1 (4): 244–250.

Erdman L, (1992). Nursing Implications of Supportive Therapies in Cancer Care, in, Clark JC, McGee RF, (eds). *Core Curriculum for Oncology Nursing,* (2nd ed). Philadelphia: WB Saunders.

Fischer D, Knobf T, (1989). *The Cancer Chemotherapy Handbook,* (3rd ed). Chicago: Year Book Medical.

Fry S, (1986). Ethical Aspects of Decision-making in the Feeding of Cancer Patients. *Seminars in Oncology Nursing.* 2 (4): 59–62.

Goodman M, Wickham R, (1984). Venous Access Devices: An Overview. *Oncology Nursing Forum.* 11 (5): 16–23.

Hagle ME, (1987). Implantable Devices for Chemotherapy: Access and Delivery. *Seminars in Oncology Nursing.* 3 (2): 96–105.

Hathorn JW, (1989). Empiric Antibiotics for Febrile Neutropenic Cancer Patients. *European Journal of Cancer and Clinical Oncology.* 25 (2): S42–S51.

Ho W, (1990). Transfusion and Aphereses of Blood Cells, in, Haskell C, (ed). *Cancer Treatment.* Philadelphia: WB Saunders, pp. 862–866.

Hughes HT, Armstrong D, Bodey GP, Feld R, et al., (1990). Guidelines for the Use of Antimicrobial Agents in Neutropenic Patients with Unexplained Fever. *Journal of Infectious Diseases.* 161: 381–396.

Jassak PF, Godwin J, (1991). Blood Component Therapy, in, Baird SB, McCorkle R, Grant M, (eds). *Cancer Nursing: A Comprehensive Textbook.* Philadephia: WB Saunders, pp. 370–384.

Klemm P, Hubbard S, (1990). Infection, in, Groenwald SL, Frogge MH, Goodman M, Yarbro CH, (eds). *Cancer Nursing Principles and Practice,* (2nd ed). Boston: Jones and Bartlett, pp. 442–466.

Leib PA, Hurting JB, (1985). Epidural and Intrathecal Narcotics for Pain Management. *Heart and Lung.* 14 (2): 164–174.

Lokich JJ, et al., (1985). Complications and Management of Implanted Venous Access Catheters. *Journal of Clinical Oncology.* 3: 710–717.

Mayer KH, DeTorres OH, (1985). Current Guidelines on the Use of Antibacterial Drugs in Patients with Malignancies. *Drugs.* 29: 262–279.

McGuire D, Braine H, (1990). Blood Component Therapy. *Seminars in Oncology Nursing.* 6 (2): 90–172.

McNally JC, Stair J, (1991). Potential for Infection, in, McNally JC, Somerville ET, Miaskowski C, Rostad M, (eds). *Guidelines for Oncology Nursing Practice,* (2nd ed). Philadelphia: WB Saunders, pp. 191–201.

Mioduszewski J, Zarbo AG, (1987). Ambulatory Infusion Pumps: A Practical View at an Alternative Approach. *Seminars in Oncology Nursing.* 3 (2): 106–111.

Moore CL, Erikson K, Yanis LB, (1986). Nursing Care and Management of Venous Access Ports. *Oncology Nursing Forum.* 13 (3): 35–39.

Oncology Nursing Society, (1989). *Access Device Guidelines, Modules I, Catheters.* Pittsburgh: Oncology Nursing Society.

Oncology Nursing Society, (1989). *Access Device Guidelines, Module II, Implanted Ports and Reservoirs.* Pittsburgh: Oncology Nursing Society.

Oncology Nursing Society, (1990). *Venous Access Guidelines, Module III, Pumps.* Pittsburgh: Oncology Nursing Society.

Rostad ME, (1990). Management of Myelosuppression in the Patient with Cancer. *Oncology Nursing Forum,*(supp). 17 (1): 4–8.

Rostad M, (1992). Nursing Implications of Supportive Procedures in Cancer Care, in, Clark JC, McGee RF, (eds). *Core Curriculum for Oncology Nursing,* (2nd ed). Philadelphia: WB Saunders.

Szeluga D, Groenwald SL, Sullivan DK, (1990). Nutritional Disturbances, in, Groenwald SL, Frogge MH, Goodman M, Yarbro CH, (eds). *Cancer Nursing Principles and Practice,* (2nd ed). Boston: Jones and Bartlett, pp. 495–519.

Von Ruemeling R, MacDonald M, Langevin T, Buchwald H, Hrushesky W, (1986). Chemotherapy via Implanted Infusion Pump: New Perspectives for Delivery of Long Term Continuous Treatment. *Oncology Nursing Forum.* 13 (2): 17–24.

Wade JC, (1989). Antibiotic Therapy for the Febrile Granulocytopenic Cancer Patient: Combination Therapy versus Monotherapy. *Review of Infectious Diseases.* 11 (7): S1572–S1581.

Wenzel RP, (1987). *Prevention and Control of Nosocomial Infections.* Baltimore: Williams and Wilkins.

12 Characteristics of Major Cancers

Lung
Lisa Potanovich and Leslie B. Tyson

Breast
Nina M. Entrekin

Genitourinary
Karen L. Fitz Adelman

Reproductive
Marie Flannery

Gastro-intestinal
Roberta Anne Strohl

Hematologic and Lymphatic Systems
Cathy Mazzone

Skin
Alice J. Longman

Head and Neck
Leonita H. Cutright

Neurologic
Betty M. Owens

Sarcoma
Tracy Kresek

HIV Infection and AIDS
James P. Halloran

Lung
Lisa Potanovich and Leslie B. Tyson

Select the BEST answer for all of the following questions:

1. A 66-year-old male patient is seen in the outpatient setting complaining of increasing dyspnea. Significant history and physical findings are
   1. 40 pack/years of unfiltered cigarette smoking
   2. urban dweller
   3. diagnosis of chronic bronchitis
   4. increasing fatigue with exertion
   5. smoker's cough in the morning with expectoration
   6. decreased breath sounds and scattered wheezes

   The most likely diagnosis includes all of the following **EXCEPT**
   A. lung cancer.
   B. emphysema.
   C. atelectasis.
   D. normal physiological changes with aging.

1. *Answer:* **C**

    Rationale: Presents a very typical clinical picture for lung cancer that is frequently missed because the health professional assumes the problem is due to physical problems other than cancer.

2.   Mr. S is about to be discharged from the hospital following removal of the right middle lobe for non-small cell lung cancer. He complains of shortness of breath when ambulating and is coughing up small amounts of thick, white sputum since the surgery. Management at home should be aimed at all of the following **EXCEPT**

   A.   encouraging use of bronchodilators as ordered by the physician.
   B.   encouraging good pulmonary toilet such as deep-breathing exercises and coughing exercises.
   C.   encouraging rest and taking two acetaminophen if a fever develops (greater than 101°F).
   D.   encouraging the use of pain medication to facilitate mobility.

3.   Mrs. S has completed a course of radiotherapy following resection of a stage II non-small cell lung cancer. Her tumor is under control at this time. Her most common complaint is constant fatigue. All of the following describe good advice **EXCEPT**

   A.   explaining to the patient that fatigue is expected temporarily following radiation therapy.
   B.   requiring a progressive ambulation plan with scheduled rest periods as needed.
   C.   suggesting that the patient maintain activities that are important to her.
   D.   encouraging the patient to return to her work schedule.

4.   Mr. S has just been discharged from the hospital following a right middle lobectomy for lung cancer. Since his diagnosis he has quit smoking, but finds it difficult to adapt to a non-smoking lifestyle. Which of the following describes good advice for Mr. S?

   A.   There is no reason to stop smoking now; the tumor has been removed. The worst of the danger is over.
   B.   Continue to encourage Mr. S not to smoke.
   C.   Encourage Mr. S to gradually decrease the number of cigarettes he smokes each day.
   D.   Encourage Mr. S to be around smokers when he has the urge for a cigarette.

5.   A 53-year-old woman has stage I lung cancer and had a left upper lobectomy. Which one of the following actions should be part of the plan of care?

   A.   Limit activity during hospitalization.
   B.   Promote good pulmonary toilet.
   C.   Withhold pain medication before breathing exercises.
   D.   Limit visitors to prevent infection.

6.   A 44-year-old woman with non-small cell lung cancer is admitted to the hospital for cisplatin therapy. The post-treatment plan of care should include which of the following?

   A.   Monitor intake and output.
   B.   Check post-treatment WBC.
   C.   Hold antiemetic if diarrhea occurs.
   D.   Observe for hair loss.

2. *Answer:* **C**

    Rationale: Postoperatively, patients require good pulmonary toilet to prevent infection and to promote adequate ventilation. The use of pain medicine, as well as bronchodilators, may be necessary to facilitate this. A postoperative fever is usually an indication of infection or pneumonia and requires immediate notification of the physician.

3. *Answer:* **D**

    Rationale: Fatigue following radiation therapy is common for many patients and is usually temporary. It is important to encourage the patient to return to normal activities as soon as possible, but the patient should do so gradually, so as not to become discouraged.

4. *Answer:* **B**

    Rationale: While decreasing the number of cigarettes smoked each day may be helpful, the best answer is B. Continued cigarette smoking may put the patient at risk for a second cancer as well as a greater risk for infection.

5. *Answer:* **B**

    Rationale: Postoperative complications can occur if good pulmonary toilet is not implemented. Deep-breathing and coughing exercises assist in eliminating secretions. This promotes adequate gas exchange and prevents infection.

6. *Answer:* **A**

    Rationale: Cisplatin is an agent that causes nephrotoxicity. It is important to monitor renal function closely. With the additional side effect of nausea and vomiting, fluid and electrolyte imbalances can occur. Therefore, it is important to maintain strict intake and output.

7.   A 53-year-old woman is suspected of having lung cancer. Bronchoscopy was performed to confirm a diagnosis. On returning to the unit, care should include all of the following **EXCEPT**
   A.   positioning patient flat on back.
   B.   instructing patient to take nothing by mouth (NPO) until gag reflex returns.
   C.   observing for signs of laryngospasm or laryngeal edema.
   D.   collecting any sputum the patient produces.

8.   Which one of the following cancers would have the **SHORTEST** and **POOREST** prognosis?
   A.   Extensive small cell lung cancer (SCLC).
   B.   Limited small cell lung cancer.
   C.   Non-small cell lung cancer (NSCLC), stage I.
   D.   Non-small cell lung cancer, stage II.

9.   Important prognostic factors in non-small cell lung cancer include all of the following **EXCEPT**
   A.   performance status.
   B.   location of tumor.
   C.   stage of disease.
   D.   presence of systemic symptoms.

10.   Which statement is **NOT TRUE** regarding the use of radiation therapy?
   A.   Prophylactic cranial irradiation is always given to patients with adenocarcinoma of the lung.
   B.   Radiation therapy may be used palliatively to relieve symptoms of bone pain, superior vena caval obstruction, and airway compression.

   C.   Radiation is used postoperatively in patients with positive mediastinal lymph nodes.
   D.   Radiation therapy is the treatment of choice in patients with stage I non-small cell lung cancer.

11.   Mr. S was recently diagnosed with non-small cell lung cancer. Staging work-up revealed: a 6 cm lower left lobe mass, bilateral mediastinal lymph nodes, and left adrenal metastases. He has no other medical problems. His best treatment option for control of disease is
   A.   combination chemotherapy and radiation therapy.
   B.   radiotherapy to the chest.
   C.   surgical removal of the lung lesion.
   D.   surgical removal of the lung lesion followed by radiation to the chest.

12.   Surgery is **NOT** an option for patients with
   A.   limited stage small cell lung cancer.
   B.   stage I or II non-small cell lung cancer.
   C.   stage IIIA non-small cell lung cancer.
   D.   occult stage non-small cell lung cancer.

13.   An important diagnostic procedure to obtain brushings and washings in a patient with suspected lung cancer is
   A.   chest CT scan.
   B.   chest tomogram.
   C.   upper GI.
   D.   bronchoscopy.

7.   *Answer:* **A**

Rationale: After a bronchoscopy, the patient should remain on his side, either flat or in a semi-Fowler position. The patient should be instructed not to swallow and to allow the saliva to run from side of mouth until the gag reflex returns.

8.   *Answer:* **A**

Rationale: Both extensive SCLC and stage II NSCLC have a poor prognosis for survival. However, patients with SCLC will live about thirteen months, and those with NSCLC will live beyond that. Neither group will have many survivors beyond two years.

9.   *Answer:* **B**

Rationale: Location of the tumor is not an important prognostic factor. Important prognostic factors include performance status, extent of disease, weight loss greater than ten pounds in the previous six months, and elevated serum LDH.

10.   *Answer:* **D**

Rationale: Patients with stage I non-small cell lung cancer who are otherwise healthy (i.e., no contraindication to surgery) should have surgery for a curative attempt.

11.   *Answer:* **A**

Rationale: Patients are usually treated symptomatically once they have advanced disease. They may receive chemotherapy and radiation therapy for palliation.

12.   *Answer:* **A**

Rationale: Surgical resection of lung tumors offers the only chance of cure. Candidates for surgical resection include patients with occult and stage I and II non-small cell lung cancers. Occasionally, patients with *limited stage IIIA* non-small cell lung cancers are considered for surgery. Small cell lung cancer is always considered a systemic disease that responds very well to chemotherapy and radiotherapy.

13.   *Answer:* **D**

Rationale: Chest CT scans and tomograms are radiographic procedures. Bronchoscopy is a means of obtaining cells to make a diagnosis.

14. Mrs. L has recently been diagnosed with limited stage small cell lung cancer. She is now admitted for chemotherapy with cisplatin and etoposide. On admission, hematologic and biochemical parameters are sodium of 129, potassium of 4.3, chloride of 102, and carbon dioxide of 26. After vigorous intravenous hydration, Mrs. L is found to be lethargic, disoriented, and confused. Mrs. L is most likely exhibiting symptoms of
    A. hypercalcemia.
    B. syndrome of inappropriate antidiuretic hormone (SIADH).
    C. hypertrophic pulmonary osteoarthropathy.
    D. Horner's syndrome.

15. Which one of the following is **NOT** descriptive of small cell lung cancer?
    A. Rapid growth rate.
    B. Tendency to metastasize early.
    C. Most common type of lung cancer.
    D. Strongly associated with cigarette smoking.

16. Which of the following is **NOT** a frequent presenting symptom of lung cancer?
    A. Cough.
    B. Anemia.
    C. Dyspnea.
    D. Hemoptysis.

Breast

Nina M. Entrekin

Select the BEST answer for all of the following questions:

1. The majority of breast cancers occur in which area of the breast?
    A. Upper outer quadrant.
    B. Upper inner quadrant.
    C. Lower outer quadrant.
    D. Beneath the nipple/areola.

2. After breast surgery with axillary node dissection, the rationale for elevating the affected arm of the patient with the elbow at the level of the heart is to
    A. minimize tension on the suture lines.
    B. prevent fluid accumulation under skin flaps.
    C. promote venous and lymphatic drainage.
    D. promote functional recovery of the arm.

3. Which of the following risk factors for breast cancer is classified as a **PRIMARY** risk factor?
    A. Birth of first child after 30 years of age.
    B. Mother or sister has history of breast cancer.
    C. Long-term estrogen replacement therapy.
    D. History of frequent biopsies for fibrocystic disease.

4. Peau d'orange is a common sign associated with which type of breast cancer?
    A. Infiltrating ductal.
    B. Infiltrating lobular.
    C. Inflammatory.
    D. Mucinous.

14. *Answer:* **B**

Rationale: Signs and symptoms of SIADH are described. Admission sodium is borderline normal. SIADH is a known paraneoplastic syndrome associated with SCLC.

15. *Answer:* **C**

Rationale: Adenocarcinoma is the most common type of lung cancer. Cigarette smoking is more strongly correlated with epidermoid and small cell lung cancers. Small cell lung cancer has a rapid rate of growth and a tendency to metastasize early.

16. *Answer:* **B**

Rationale: The most common presenting symptoms include cough, dyspnea, and hemoptysis. Systemic symptoms such as fatigue and weight loss may also be present.

REFERENCES

Britton D, (1983). Fatigue, in, Yasko JM, (ed). *Guidelines for Cancer Care: Symptom Management.* Reston, VA: Reston Publishing Co., pp. 33–37.

Elpern EH, (1990). Lung Cancer, in, Groenwald SL, Frogge MH, Goodman M, Yarbro CH, (eds). *Cancer Nursing Principles and Practice,* (2nd ed). Boston: Jones and Bartlett. pp. 951–973.

Frank-Stromborg M, Cohen R, (1990). Assessment and Interventions for Cancer Prevention and Detection, in, Groenwald SL, Frogge MH, Goodman M, Yarbro CH, (eds). *Cancer Nursing Principles and Practice* (2nd ed). Boston: Jones and Bartlett, pp 119–160.

Griffiths MJ, Murray KH, Russo PC, (1984). Cancer of the Lung and Mediastinum, in, *Oncology Nursing. Pathophysiology, Assessment, and Intervention.* New York: Macmillan Publishing Co., pp. 184–199.

Hogan CM, (1983). Nausea and Vomiting, in, Yasko JM, (ed). *Guidelines for Cancer Care: Symptom Management.* Reston, VA: Reston Publishing Co., pp. 198–211.

Irwin M, Yasko JM, (1983). Respiratory System Dysfunction, in, *Guidelines for Cancer Care: Symptom Management.* Reston, VA: Reston Publishing Co., pp. 249–264.

Larkin M, Benson LM, (1991). Ineffective Airway Clearance, in, McNally JC, Somerville ET, Miaskowski C, Rostad M, (eds). *Guidelines for Cancer Nursing Practice,* (2nd ed). Philadelphia: WB Saunders, pp. 353–358.

Lend J, (1992). Lung Cancer, in, Clark JC, McGee RF, (eds). *Core Curriculum in Oncology Nursing,* (2nd ed). Philadelphia: WB Saunders.

Lindsey AM, (1991). Lung Cancer, in, Baird SB, McCorkle R, Grant M, (eds). *Cancer Nursing: A Comprehensive Textbook.* Philadephia: WB Saunders, pp. 452–465.

McNally JC, Somerville ET, Miaskowski C, Rostad M, (eds), (1991). Ventilation, in, *Guidelines for Oncology Nursing Practice,* (2nd ed). Philadelphia: WB Saunders. pp. 351–384.

Minna JD, Pass H, Glatstein E, Ihde D, (1989). Cancer of the Lung, in, Devita VT, Hellman S, Rosenberg S, (eds). *Cancer Principles and Practice of Oncology,* (3rd ed). Philadelphia: JB Lippincott, pp. 591–705.

O'Connell J, Kris MG, Gralla RJ, et al., (1986). Frequency and Prognostic Importance of Pretreatment Clinical Characteristics in Patients with Advanced Non-Small Cell Lung Cancer Treated with Combination Chemotherapy. *Journal of Clinical Oncology.* 4: 1604–1614.

Polomano R, McEvay MD, (1991). Nursing Management of Persons with Progressive Disease: Prototype—Lung Cancer, in, Baird SB, McCorkle R, Grant M, (eds). *Cancer Nursing: A Comprehensive Textbook.* Philadelphia: WB Saunders, pp. 699–707.

Yarbro CH, Cantril C, Frogge MH, et al., (1988). *Oncology: Programmed Modules for Nurses Vol. 3, Types of Cancer, Part A.* New York: LP Communications Inc.

Breast

1. *Answer:* **A**

Rationale: 48% of malignant tumors occur in the upper outer quadrant of the breast.

2. *Answer:* **C**

Rationale: Elevating the arm uses gravity to promote venous return and drainage of lymph.

3. *Answer:* **B**

Rationale: Primary risk factors are female, age over 45, personal history of breast cancer, and family history of breast cancer.

4. *Answer:* **C**

Rationale: Peau d'orange is an ominous sign associated with inflammatory breast cancer.

5.   Ultrasonography is used in the diagnosis of breast cancer to
   A.   supplement mammography in evaluating dense breast tissue.
   B.   distinguish between fluid-filled cysts and solid masses.
   C.   substitute for mammography when breast compression is inadequate.
   D.   distinguish between benign and malignant lesions.

6.   When a suspicious area is seen on a mammogram but is not palpable on clinical exam, an appropriate diagnostic procedure is:
   A.   fine needle aspiration.
   B.   needle core biopsy.
   C.   excisional biopsy.
   D.   needle localization.

7.   The breast cancer patient with the **LEAST** favorable prognosis would be the one whose estrogen receptor (ER) and progesterone receptor (PR) results are
   A.   ER+, PR+.
   B.   ER+, PR−.
   C.   ER−, PR+.
   D.   ER−, PR−.

8.   The patient who is the best candidate for hormonal manipulation in the presence of breast cancer metastases is the woman whose estrogen receptor (ER) and progesterone receptor (PR) results are:
   A.   ER+, PR+.
   B.   ER+, PR−.
   C.   ER−, PR+.
   D.   ER−, PR−.

9.   Ms. J has had breast surgery with axillary node dissection. Discharge instructions for the care of her affected arm might include all of the following **EXCEPT**:
   A.   wear protective gloves when gardening.
   B.   carry heavy articles with the unaffected arm.
   C.   apply ice to the arm to reduce swelling.
   D.   avoid injections of any kind in this arm.

10.   The single **MOST IMPORTANT** prognostic indicator of survival of breast cancer is
   A.   size of primary tumor.
   B.   invasiveness of tumor.
   C.   number of positive axillary nodes.
   D.   high S-phase DNA fraction.

11.   Which of the following is the most common metastatic site for breast cancer?
   A.   Lung.
   B.   Liver.
   C.   Brain.
   D.   Bone.

12.   During the first twenty-four hours after breast surgery, an appropriate level of exercise for the patient would be
   A.   brushing own hair and teeth.
   B.   squeezing a soft rubber ball.
   C.   immobilizing affected arm in sling.
   D.   rotating shoulder through 180°.

13.   A volunteer organization specifically oriented to provide support to the breast cancer patient is
   A.   ACS/Reach to Recovery.
   B.   Encore.
   C.   Y-ME.
   D.   All of the above.

14.   Ms. Y is a 32-year-old breast cancer patient who is concerned about future pregnancy. The nurse's response to Ms. Y's question is based on the understanding that
   A.   infertility after chemotherapy is a significant barrier.
   B.   hormonal changes of pregnancy increase risk of recurrence.
   C.   pregnancy should be delayed for two years after treatment.
   D.   the risk of fetal anomalies and stillbirths is increased after treatment.

15.   Education of the daughters and sisters of a woman with breast cancer should include
   A.   breast self-exam.
   B.   mammography recommendations.
   C.   annual physical exam.
   D.   all of the above.

5. *Answer:* **B**

Rationale: Ultrasonography is 95% accurate in identifying cystic versus solid masses. Responses A and D are true of CAT scans.

6. *Answer:* **D**

Rationale: Fine needle aspiration, needle core biopsy and excisional biopsy, all require that the surgeon be able to palpate/locate the tissue to be removed for microscopic exam.

7. *Answer:* **D**

Rationale: Patients whose breast tumors are estrogen and progesterone receptor negative (ER−, PR−) have a higher risk for aggressive disease with early metastasis and, thus, a poorer prognosis.

8. *Answer:* **A**

Rationale: Hormonal manipulation produces a less than 10% response rate in ER−, PR− tumors and an over 70% response rate if the tumor is ER+, PR+.

9. *Answer:* **C**

Rationale: The affected hand and arm should not be exposed to extremes of temperature.

10. *Answer:* **C**

Rationale: While several factors predict likelihood of recurrence, all sources agree that the most important prognosticator is the degree of nodal involvement.

11. *Answer:* **D**

Rationale: Metastases in breast cancer occur in the following frequencies: bone, 71%; lung, 69%; liver, 65%; and brain, 20%.

12. *Answer:* **B**

Rationale: Flexion and extension exercises promote adequate venous drainage of the arm and minimize tension on the suture line. Range of motion exercises are usually begun on the second to third day at the surgeon's discretion.

13. *Answer:* **D**

Rationale: Reach to Recovery, sponsored by the American Cancer Society since 1969, is one of the best known self-help groups. Encore is a program offered by the YWCA that provides exercise programs and support groups for women post-breast cancer surgery. Y-ME, founded by two mastectomy patients in 1978 in Illinois, is the largest breast cancer support program in the U.S.

14. *Answer:* **C**

Rationale: Risk of recurrence is greatest in the first two years after diagnosis. Deferral of pregnancy for two years after treatment is therefore recommended.

15. *Answer:* **D**

Rationale: Daughters and sisters of a woman with breast cancer are at increased risk of developing the disease and should be educated in early detection activities.

REFERENCES

Coleman CM, Crane R, (1991). Knowledge Deficit Related to Prevention and Early Detection of Breast Cancer, in, McNally JC, Somerville ET, Miaskowski C, Rostad M, (eds). *Guidelines for Oncology Nursing Practice*, (2nd ed). Philadelphia: WB Saunders, pp. 6–11.

Entrekin N, (1992). Breast Cancer, in, Clark JC, McGee RF, (eds). *Core Curriculum for Oncology Nursing*, (2nd ed). Philadelphia: WB Saunders.

Frank-Stromborg M, Savela B, (1990). Yellow Pages for the Cancer Nurse, in, Groenwald SL, Frogge MH, Goodman M, Yarbro CH, (eds). *Cancer Nursing Principles and Practice*, (2nd ed). Boston: Jones and Bartlett, pp. 1281–1308.

Goodman M, Harte N, (1990). Breast Cancer, in, Groenwald SL, Frogge MH, Goodman M, Yarbro CH, (eds). *Cancer Nursing Principles and Practice*, (2nd ed). Boston: Jones and Bartlett, pp. 722–750.

Hassey KM, (1988). Pregnancy and Parenthood after Treatment for Breast Cancer. *Oncology Nursing Forum.* 15 (4): 439–444.

Knobf MT, (1991). Breast Cancer, in, Baird SB, McCorkle R, Grant M, (eds). *Cancer Nursing: A Comprehensive Textbook.* Philadelphia: WB Saunders, pp. 425–451.

Reiss M, (1989). Prognostic Factors in Primary Breast Cancer. *Connecticut Medicine.* 53: 565–571.

Genitourinary

Karen L. Fitz Adelman

Select the BEST answer for all of the following questions:

1. A 62-year-old black male developed an acute onset of urinary retention, constipation, and pain in his back and pelvis radiating to his hips. His diagnostic work-up should include which of the following?
   - A. PSA.
   - B. Cystoscopy.
   - C. MRI of the brain.
   - D. Lower GI series.

2. Mr. D is admitted to the hospital for a radical retropubic prostatectomy and lymphadenectomy. When Mr. D asks if he will be permanently impotent after this surgery, the nurse's best response would be:
   - A. "It is too soon to know the outcome. Every patient is different."
   - B. "Ninety to one hundred percent of patients have erectile and ejaculatory impotence."
   - C. "Many patients only have a temporary impotence."
   - D. "Don't worry. New prosthetic devices are available."

3. When choosing an ostomy appliance for your patient, which of the following should be considered?
   - A. Character of patient's abdomen.
   - B. Location of stoma.
   - C. Character of stoma.
   - D. All of the above.

4. Mrs. J has just undergone a cystectomy for bladder cancer and has an ileal conduit. As part of patient teaching, the nurse should stress
   - A. changing the ostomy appliance just before bedtime.
   - B. attaching tubing every night for drainage.
   - C. taking the appliance off to bathe.
   - D. using a permanent appliance that never needs changing.

5. Which of the following symptoms will a patient with localized prostate cancer exhibit?
   - A. Fatigue, dysuria, and severe constipation.
   - B. Slow stream, frequency, and dysuria.
   - C. Nocturia, slow stream, and severe constipation.
   - D. Myalgias, confusion, and weakness.

6. Which of the following is a **TRUE** statement regarding prognosis in testicular cancer?
   - A. Nonseminomatous germ cell tumors are easily cured because they are so radiosensitive.
   - B. One-half of patients with seminoma are cured with orchiectomy and systemic chemotherapy.
   - C. Patients with elevated tumor markers have a poorer prognosis than those with normal tumor markers, regardless of tumor stage.
   - D. Persistence of elevated tumor markers after orchiectomy is considered a false positive if other clinical staging procedures are negative.

7. Benign causes of testicular symptoms include all of the following **EXCEPT**
   - A. epididymitis.
   - B. tuberculosis (TB).
   - C. hydrocele.
   - D. non-transilluminated scrotal mass.

1. *Answer:* **A**

    Rationale: PSA is the standard tumor marker for prostatic cancer. Digital exam is the most important screening test for prostatic carcinoma. Retention and constipation are symptoms of impending spinal cord compression from invasive prostatic cancer to the spinal cord, not brain metastasis.

2. *Answer:* **B**

    Rationale: The internal pudendal artery supplying the major amount of blood to the erectile tissue is not usually damaged, but in most patients, damage does occur to the prostatic plexus (lateral surface of prostate) and other parasympathetic autonomic nerve fibers during dissection.

3. *Answer:* **D**

    Rationale: The character of the patient's abdomen and location and character of the stoma are important characteristics that determine the best type of ostomy appliance for the patient.

4. *Answer:* **B**

    Rationale: In order for the bladder to drain continuously, the conduit must be drained at night. Attaching tubing to the appliance promotes drainage and prevents leakage.

5. *Answer:* **B**

    Rationale: The key word is *localized*. Constipation would not occur unless spinal cord compression was imminent. Myalgias, confusion, and weakness are symptoms associated with hypercalcemia, which would not occur in localized disease. Thus, response B provides the correct answer.

6. *Answer:* **C**

    Rationale: Elevated markers indicate a biologically aggressive tumor. Levels should decrease when treatment is effective.

7. *Answer:* **D**

    Rationale: *All* testis masses that do not transilluminate should be suspicious for malignancy. In TB, testis involvement is seen in late disease.

8.   Mr. C, who has a mixed germ cell tumor of the testis, completed a cisplatin-based chemotherapy regimen. He was heavily premedicated with antiemetics to decrease nausea/vomiting. He complains of increased swelling in his legs and itching. His blood pressure is 200/170, pulse = 122, and respiration = 28. You notify his physician that Mr. C

A.   is having an anaphylactic reaction to the antiemetics used to control nausea and vomiting.
B.   may be experiencing tumor lysis syndrome from rapid breakdown of tumor cells.
C.   is exhibiting symptoms of renal dysfunction from cisplatin.
D.   is having an allergic reaction to the cisplatin chemotherapy.

9.   Mr. C is admitted to begin his chemotherapy for refractory testicular cancer. His treatment regimen includes Ifosfamide 1.2 gm/m^2 × 5 days. Which intervention is used to prevent hematuria?

A.   Administer mesna concomitantly with Ifosfamide.
B.   Encourage frequent voiding to prevent bladder irritation.
C.   Drink 2000 cc of fluids to flush the bladder.
D.   Hydrate with at least 2 L of IV fluids every day.

10.   A 27-year-old man is admitted for a radical orchiectomy after a painful scrotal mass was discovered. His presurgery work-up should include which of the following?

A.   Serum samples for AFP and HCG.
B.   Bone scan.
C.   CT of the chest.
D.   Serum samples for CEA.

11.   The "classic triad" of symptoms for early renal cell cancer include

A.   hematuria, weight loss, and fever.
B.   hematuria, flank pain, and palpable mass.
C.   weight loss, weakness, and anemia.
D.   flank pain, weight loss, and palpable mass.

12.   Bladder cancer is considered a cancer that can be treated with a high degree of success because

A.   transurethral resection surgery is often curative with few recurrences.
B.   at the time of diagnosis, 70% of patients have localized disease.
C.   high doses of radiation can be delivered to the pelvis without much toxicity.
D.   this is an indolent tumor that metastasizes slowly.

13.   Mr. W underwent an angio-infarction of his primary renal tumor yesterday. Now he is complaining of severe abdominal pain, nausea, vomiting, and hiccoughs. His temperature has risen to 38.8°C. The nurse should first

A.   phone the physician for blood cultures and an antipyretic order.
B.   control the severe pain with an effective narcotic.
C.   notify the physician the patient has developed post infarction syndrome.
D.   increase IV fluid rate as ordered, sponge patient, and draw blood cultures.

14.   Mrs. G underwent a thoracoabdominal radical nephrectomy for removal of a 15 x 15 cm primary renal mass. Several days later, while sitting in a chair, Mrs. G commented, "It's harder for me to take a deep breath today. I just can't seem to get enough air." Yesterday, the surgeons removed both chest tubes. Her temperature this morning was 37.9°C and BP was 120/70. Breath sounds are decreased bilaterally. Which complication is most likely?

A.   Pulmonary emboli.
B.   Pneumonia.
C.   Postsurgery anemia
D.   Pneumothorax.

8. *Answer:* **C**

Rationale: Cisplatin is a nephrotoxic chemotherapeutic agent. Early signs and symptoms of urinary system dysfunction include lethargy, restlessness, insomnia, hypertension, increased rate and depth of respiration, dependent edema, pruritus, anorexia, nausea and vomiting, and diarrhea.

9. *Answer:* **A**

Rationale: Mesna administration is the only intervention that will decrease chance of hematuria to <6%. The other interventions alone, without mesna, do not effectively prevent hematuria.

10. *Answer:* **A**

Rationale: AFP and HCG are tumor markers specific for testicular cancer.

11. *Answer:* **C**

Rationale: This triad is present in 33% of patients at presentation with early disease, as compared to 9% of patients who present with the advanced triad of symptoms—hematuria, flank pain, and palpable mass.

12. *Answer:* **B**

Rationale: Only 7% of patients have evidence of metastasis at time of diagnosis; 75% of patients have symptoms of hematuria or bladder irritation that lead to early diagnosis. Early treatment allows a greater degree of treatment success.

13. *Answer:* **C**

Rationale: Post infarction syndrome lasts thirty-six to seventy-two hours after the embolization procedure. Pain must be controlled with narcotics, IV fluids and antiemetics administered for vomiting, fever controlled, and neurovascular signs monitored.

14. *Answer:* **D**

Rationale: A tumor this large has a good possibility of invading the diaphragm, causing a pneumothorax. This is often controlled with chest tubes if chest x-ray shows a 25% or greater pneumothorax at the time of surgery. The patient should be observed once the chest tubes are removed. Pleural fluid can reaccumulate. Pulmonary emboli result in more air hunger, pneumonia, and a higher fever.

REFERENCES

Britton D, Yasko J, (1983). Hypercalcemia, in, Yasko J, (ed). *Guidelines for Cancer Care: Symptom Management.* Reston, VA: Reston Publishing Co., pp. 336–342.

Cushman K, (1991). Knowledge Deficit Related to Prevention and Early Detection of Bladder Cancer, in, McNally JC, Somerville ET, Miaskowski C, Rostad M, (eds). *Guidelines for Oncology Nursing Practice*, (2nd ed). Philadelphia: WB Saunders, pp. 3–5.

Fitz K, (1990). *The Administration of Ifosfamide and Mesna.* Monograph, Bristol Myers-Squibb.

Lind JM, Nakao SL, (1990). Urologic and Male Genital Cancers, in, Groenwald SL, Frogge MH, Goodman M, Yarbro CH, (eds). *Cancer Nursing Principles and Practice*, (2nd ed). Boston: Jones and Bartlett, pp. 1026–1076.

Lind L, (1992). Genitourinary Cancer, in, Clark JC, McGee RF, (eds). *Core Curriculum for Oncology Nursing*, (2nd ed). Philadelphia: WB Saunders.

Lind J, Irwin RJ, (1991). Genitourinary Cancers, in, Baird SB, McCorkle R, Grant M, (eds). *Cancer Nursing: A Comprehensive Textbook.* Philadelphia: WB Saunders, pp. 466–484.

Hubbard S, Jenkins J, (1983). An Overview of Current Concepts in the Management of Patients with Testicular Tumors of Germ Cell Origin. Part I and II. *Cancer Nursing.* 6 (1): 39–47, 6 (2): 125–139.

Martin JC, (1991). Knowledge Deficit Related to Prevention and Early Detection of Prostate Cancer, in, McNally JC, Somerville ET, Miaskowski C, Rostad M, (eds). *Guidelines for Oncology Nursing Practice*, (2nd ed). Philadelphia: WB Saunders, pp. 32–34.

Martin, JP, (1991). Knowledge Deficit Related to Prevention and Early Detection of Testicular Cancer, in, McNally JC, Somerville ET, Miaskowski C, Rostad M, (eds). *Guidelines for Oncology Nursing Practice*, (2nd ed). Philadelphia: WB Saunders, pp. 44–46.

McNally JC, Somerville ET, Miaskowski C, Rostad M, (eds), (1991). Elimination, in, *Guidelines for Oncology Nursing Practice*, (2nd ed). Philadelphia: WB Saunders. pp. 295–336.

Sella A, Logothetis CJ, Fitz K, et al., (1990). Increased Response Rate of α-Interferon (Roferon) Combined with Chemotherapy: 5-Fluorouracil, Mitomycin-C in Patients with Metastatic Renal Cell Carcinoma, in, *Combining Biological Response Modifiers with Cytoxics in the Treatment of Cancer: Developing a Rational Approach to New Therapy.* National Cancer Institute, March, p. 4.

Reproductive
Marie Flannery

Select the BEST answer for all of the following questions:

1. You have been asked to present an in-service education program to nurses on risk factors for cervical cancer. You plan to include a discussion of all the following factors **EXCEPT**
    A. multiple sexual partners.
    B. sexual intercourse at an early age.
    C. number of pregnancies.
    D. human papilloma virus (HPV).

2. The *most common* presenting symptom of endometrial cancer is
    A. acute abdominal pain.
    B. increased abdominal girth.
    C. abnormal vaginal bleeding.
    D. milky vaginal drainage.

3. A patient is receiving cisplatin and cyclophosphamide for treatment of ovarian cancer. In developing her nursing care plan, you would include assessment of all of the following side effects **EXCEPT**
    A. alopecia.
    B. stomatitis.
    C. nausea and vomiting.
    D. neuropathies.

4. You have an opportunity to examine survivorship issues in a long-term follow-up clinic for patients with testicular cancer. In developing an assessment tool, which of the following areas would **NOT** logically be included?
    A. School-age learning deficits.
    B. Reemployment issues.
    C. Insurance coverage.
    D. Occurrence of second malignancies.

5. A patient had a "suspicious" Pap smear and is now admitted for a diagnostic workup. She is scheduled for a cystoscopy and proctosigmoidoscopy. In explaining why these procedures are necessary, you emphasize that the test results
    A. will determine if the cancer has spread to adjacent organs.
    B. are used primarily to rule out other types of cancer.
    C. will determine how much surgery will be necessary.
    D. will determine the size of the radiation field.

6. As part of your nursing interventions to assist the patient with testicular cancer in adapting to his disease, you initiate a conversation about the possibility of sperm banking prior to beginning chemotherapy. Which of the following information would you discuss?
    A. Patients are fertile prior to treatment beginning.
    B. Insurance carriers pay for sperm banking.
    C. Impotence is common after treatment.
    D. Infertility is common after treatment.

7. You are caring for a woman who has just been diagnosed with endometrial cancer. She tells you she does not understand how she can have cancer when her Pap smear was negative eight months ago. Which one of the following is the most appropriate response?
    A. Many Pap smears are not interpreted correctly.
    B. Endometrial cancer may develop in a very short time.
    C. The Pap specimen may have been obtained incorrectly.
    D. Pap smears do not commonly detect endometrial cancer.

1. *Answer:* **C**

   Rationale: Pregnancy or the absence of pregnancy is not a risk factor in cervical cancer. A history of HPV, early intercourse, and multiple partners are the significant influencing factors.

2. *Answer:* **C**

   Rationale: Abdominal discomfort and increasing girth are significant symptoms of ovarian cancer. Milky vaginal drainage may occur with cervical cancer. Twenty percent of postmenopausal bleeding is related to endometrial cancer.

3. *Answer:* **B**

   Rationale: Cisplatin and cyclophosphamide are the two most commonly used drugs in the management of ovarian cancer. Both drugs have a low potential for causing stomatitis.

4. *Answer:* **A**

   Rationale: Learning deficits are a common survivorship issue for childhood

cancers. Patients with testicular cancer are generally past school age years at time of diagnosis.

5. *Answer:* **A**

   Rationale: These diagnostic tests are commonly used for all the reasons listed. However, the primary purpose in cervical cancer is to determine any local extension.

6. *Answer:* **D**

   Rationale: Requires knowledge of infertility versus impotence in relation to sterility. Infertility may be present prior to treatment and health insurance coverage for sperm banking is not always assured.

7. *Answer:* **D**

   Rationale: Exfoliated malignant cells from the endometrium are rarely picked up on a cervical sampling (the Pap test). Pap smear is a *screening* test for cervical intraepithelial neoplasias or invasive cervical cancer.

8.   A patient you are caring for has completed radiation therapy for cervical cancer. You are teaching her about the use of a vaginal dilator to prevent vaginal stenosis. You would include all of the following instructions **EXCEPT**
   A.   use three to five times a week.
   B.   use a water-based lubricant.
   C.   use for ten to twenty minutes.
   D.   sexual intercourse is not a substitute.

9.   You are caring for a patient who is three months postop from a radical hysterectomy as curative treatment for cervical cancer. You are having a conversation about the resumption of sexual relations. You would include all of the following recommendations **EXCEPT**
   A.   waiting until all discomfort resolves with healing.
   B.   use a water-based lubricant for vaginal moisture.
   C.   experiment with alternate coital positions for increased comfort.
   D.   discuss fears and concerns with her spouse.

10.   Factors that are commonly associated with the prognosis of endometrial cancer include all of the following **EXCEPT**
   A.   anatomic stage of disease.
   B.   cellular histology and differentiation.
   C.   depth of myometrial invasion.
   D.   presence or absence of ascites.

11.   A woman presents with advanced ovarian cancer. All of the following may be common findings **EXCEPT**
   A.   abdominal mass.
   B.   ascites.
   C.   pleural effusion.
   D.   vaginal hemorrhage.

12.   A patient with testicular cancer is beginning a course of external beam-radiation therapy to the lungs. He has previously received four cycles of chemotherapy: cisplatin, etoposide and bleomycin. In developing your nursing care plan, a priority in your assessment is
   A.   gastrointestinal distress.
   B.   respiratory distress.
   C.   myelosuppression.
   D.   fatigue.

13.   The wife of a patient with testicular cancer stops you in the hall. Her husband is receiving his first cycle of chemotherapy. She tells you she doesn't know what she'll do when he dies. In forming your response, you remember that the prognosis for testicular cancer is
   A.   highly variable depending on stage.
   B.   highly variable depending on histology.
   C.   excellent and considered a curable disease.
   D.   less than a 70% survival rate.

8. *Answer:* **D**

Rationale: Use of a vaginal dilator is necessary if regular sexual intercourse is not maintained. Specific instructions on duration and frequency need to be provided. Use of a water-based lubricant will increase comfort. Sexual activity on a regular basis is acceptable as an alternative for preventing vaginal stenosis.

9. *Answer:* **A**

Rationale: Some discomfort with intercourse may occur in the first efforts at intercourse after surgery. However, it can be minimized by vaginal lubrication, positions with less deep penetration, and a sensitive, well-informed partner.

10. *Answer:* **D**

Rationale: Stage, histology, differentiation, and depth of invasion are prognostic factors for endometrial cancer. Ascites is rare in this disease, but a common presenting symptom in ovarian cancer.

11. *Answer:* **D**

Rationale: Vaginal hemorrhage is an indicator of endometrial or cervical cancer. It is not associated with ovarian cancer as are the other symptoms.

12. *Answer:* **B**

Rationale: Previous treatment with bleomycin can increase the risk of pulmonary fibrosis. All of these symptoms are side effects of radiation therapy, but respiratory distress would be the highest priority.

13. *Answer:* **C**

Rationale: Testicular cancer is a model for a curable solid tumor.

14. In a patient with ovarian cancer, which symptom would **NOT** automatically arouse the nurse's suspicion for the presence of recurrent disease?

    A. Increased abdominal girth.
    B. Confusion.
    C. Weight loss.
    D. Anorexia.

15. As part of the diagnostic workup for testicular cancer, laboratory tests of serum tumor markers, alpha fetoprotein (AFP) and beta human chorionic gonadotropin (BHCG), are often conducted to establish histology. AFP and BHCG levels are usually elevated in most

    A. seminomas.
    B. nonseminomas.
    C. both seminomas and nonseminomas.
    D. neither seminomas nor nonseminomas.

14. *Answer:* **B**

Rationale: Ovarian cancer usually recurs locally, and symptoms are often related to malabsorption or abdominal problems. Confusion, a common symptom of brain metastasis, is not a common finding in ovarian cancer.

15. *Answer:* **B**

Rationale: AFP and BHCG are elevated in nonseminomas. Pure seminomas may have elevated BHCG, but AFP is not elevated.

REFERENCES

Beecham JB, Angel C, (1987). Gynecologic Oncology, in, Rosenthal S, Carrigan J, Smith B, (eds). *Medical Care of the Oncology Patient*. Philadelphia: WB Saunders, pp. 274–290.

Berk JS, Hacker NF, (1989). *Practical Gynecologic Oncology*. Baltimore: Williams and Wilkins.

Brown JK, Hogan CM, (1990). Chemotherapy, in, Groenwald SL, Frogge MH, Goodman M, Yarbro CH, (eds). *Cancer Nursing Principles and Practice,* (2nd ed). Boston: Jones and Bartlett, pp. 230–283.

Clark JC, (1991). Mucous Membrane Integrity, Impairment of, Related to Vaginal Changes, in, McNally JC, Somerville ET, Miaskowski C, Rostad M, (eds). *Guidelines for Oncology Nursing Practice,* (2nd ed). Philadelphia: WB Saunders, pp. 248–251.

Einhorn L, (1990). Treatment of Testicular Cancer: A New and Improved Model. *Journal of Clinical Oncology*. 8: 1777–1781.

Eriksson JA, Walczak JR, (1990). Ovarian Cancer. *Seminars in Oncology Nursing*. 6 (3): 214–227.

Fanslair J, (1991). Knowledge Deficit Related to Prevention and Early Detection of Cervical and Uterine (Endometrial) Cancer, in, McNally JC, Somerville ET, Miaskowski C, Rostad M, (eds). *Guidelines for Oncology Nursing Practice,* (2nd ed). Philadelphia: WB Saunders, pp. 12–16.

Flannery M, (1992). Reproductive Cancers, in, Clark JC, McGee RF, (eds). *Core Curriculum in Oncology Nursing,* (2nd ed). Philadelphia: WB Saunders.

Gelbard S, (1991). Knowledge Deficit Related to Contraception, in, McNally JC, Somerville ET, Miaskowski C, Rostad M, (eds). *Guidelines for Oncology Nursing Practice,* (2nd ed). Philadelphia: WB Saunders, pp. 95–96.

Glasgow M, Halfin V, Althausen A, (1987). Sexual Response and Cancer. *CA*. 37 (6): 322–332.

Hubbard JL, Holcombe JK, (1990). Cancer of the Endometrium. *Seminars in Oncology Nursing*. 6 (3): 207.

Krebs LU, (1990). Sexual and Reproductive Dysfunction, in, Groenwald SL, Frogge MH, Goodman M, Yarbro CH, (eds). *Cancer Nursing Principles and Practice,* (2nd ed). Boston: Jones and Bartlett, pp. 563–580.

Lamb MA, (1991). Alterations in Sexuality and Sexual Functioning, in, Baird SB, McCorkle R, Grant M, (eds). *Cancer Nursing: A Comprehensive Textbook*. Philadelphia: WB Saunders, pp. 831–849.

Lind JM, Nakao S, (1990). Urologic and Male Genital Cancers, in, Groenwald SL, Frogge MH, Goodman M, Yarbro CH, (eds). *Cancer Nursing Principles and Practice,* (2nd ed). Boston: Jones and Bartlett, pp. 1026–1076.

Martin JP, (1991). Knowledge Deficit Related to Prevention and Early Detection of Testicular Cancer, in, McNally JC, Somerville ET, Miaskowski C, Rostad M, (eds). *Guidelines for Oncology Nursing Practice*, (2nd ed). Philadelphia: WB Saunders, pp. 44–46.

Martin LK, Braly PS, (1991). Gynecologic Cancers, in, Baird SB, McCorkle R, Grant M, (eds). *Cancer Nursing: A Comprehensive Textbook*. Philadephia: WB Saunders, pp. 502–535.

McNally JC, Somerville ET, Miaskowski C, Rostad M, (eds). (1991). Sexuality, in, *Guidelines for Oncology Nursing Practice*, (2nd ed). Philadelphia: WB Saunders, pp. 337–350.

Otte DM, (1990). Gynecologic Cancers, in, Groenwald SL, Frogge MH, Goodman M, Yarbro CH, (eds). *Cancer Nursing Principles and Practice,* (2nd ed). Boston: Jones and Bartlett, pp. 845–888.

Richards S, Hiratyka S, (1986). Vaginal Dilation Post Pelvic Irradiation: A Patient Education Tool. *Oncology Nursing Forum*. 13: 89-91.

Riekier P, Fitzgerald E, Kalish L, (1990). Adaptive Behavioral Responses to Potential Infertility Among Survivors of Testicular Cancer. *Journal of Clinical Oncology*. 8: 347–355.

Schover L, (1988). *Sexuality and Cancer*. New York: American Cancer Society.

Somner K, Brockmann WP, Hubner K, (1990). Treatment Results and Acute and Late Toxicity of Radiation Therapy for Testicular Seminoma. *Cancer*. 66: 259–263.

Thompson LJ, (1990). Cancer of the Cervix. *Seminars in Oncology Nursing*. 6 (3): 190–192.

Welch-McCaffery D, Leigh S, Loescher L, Hoffman B, (1990). Psychosocial Dimensions: Issues in Survivorship, in, Groenwald SL, Frogge MH, Goodman M, Yarbro CH, (eds). *Cancer Nursing Principles and Practice*, (2nd ed). Boston: Jones and Bartlett, pp. 373–382.

Gastro-intestinal
Roberta Anne Strohl

Select the BEST answer for all of the following questions:

1. The most common gastrointestinal cancer is
   A. stomach.
   B. liver.
   C. colorectal.
   D. pancreas.

2. In which region does obstruction of the bowel occur most commonly in colon cancer?
   A. Sigmoid.
   B. Ascending.
   C. Transverse.
   D. Descending.

3. Which tumor marker has been useful in monitoring for recurrence of colorectal cancer?
   A. AFP.
   B. HCG.
   C. CEA.
   D. OAF.

4. The most common presenting symptom in pancreatic cancer is
   A. nausea.
   B. pain.
   C. headache.
   D. weight loss.

5. The most effective screening method for colorectal cancer is
   A. barium enema.
   B. stool hemocult.
   C. colonoscopy.
   D. rectal exam.

6. The chemotherapeutic regimen recommended for Dukes' B and C colon cancer includes
   A. methotrexate and 5-FU.
   B. CBDCA and bleomycin.
   C. MOPP.
   D. levamisole and 5-FU.

7. The most common side effect in patients receiving radiation therapy for colorectal cancer is
   A. nausea.
   B. diarrhea.
   C. bone marrow depression.
   D. intestinal obstruction.

8. The primary therapy for potentially curable colorectal cancer is
   A. immunotherapy.
   B. radiation.
   C. surgery.
   D. chemotherapy.

9. The risk of lymph node metastases in colon cancer is correlated with which characteristic of the primary tumor?
   A. Size.
   B. Location.
   C. Grade.
   D. Ulceration.

10. The critical anatomical structure that limits the radiation dose in treating colon cancer is the
    A. small bowel.
    B. large intestine.
    C. abdominal aorta.
    D. rectum.

11. The distal segment of the colon that is sutured to the abdominal wall in a double-barrel colostomy is also known as a
    A. loop colostomy.
    B. fascial bridge.
    C. mucous fistula.
    D. distal colostomy.

12. The surgical procedure for pancreatic cancer that involves a pancreatojejunostomy is also known as the
    A. Billroth procedure.
    B. McBurney procedure.
    C. Halstead procedure.
    D. Whipple procedure.

1. *Answer:* **C**

    Rationale: 110,000 new cases of cancer of the large intestine and 45,000 cases of cancer of the rectum were reported in 1990.

2. *Answer:* **A**

    Rationale: The obstruction is usually the result of the type of tumors characteristic of this area which cause a decrease in the size of the bowel lumen.

3. *Answer:* **C**

    Rationale: Carcinoembryonic antigen (CEA) is generally elevated in persons with colon cancer. It is used to monitor the efficacy of treatment.

4. *Answer:* **B**

    Rationale: Tumors of the pancreas grow rapidly without overt signs and symptoms of the pathology. Pain is often the presenting symptom.

5. *Answer:* **C**

    Rationale: This test provides the most complete visualization of the colon.

6. *Answer:* **D**

    Rationale: Research has shown increased survival with this drug combination.

7. *Answer:* **B**

    Rationale: The rapid mitotic rate of GI mucosa cells results in sensitivity to radiation.

8. *Answer:* **C**

    Rationale: The rate and pattern of growth of colorectal cancer makes excision of local disease the treatment of choice.

9. *Answer:* **C**

    Rationale: Increase in grade indicates a more anaplastic tumor with a greater likelihood of metastases.

10. *Answer:* **A**

    Rationale: The small bowel tolerates only low doses of radiation therapy with conventional techniques.

11. *Answer:* **C**

    Rationale: The defunctionalized segment of colon is not removed and continues to produce mucous. The proximal bowel contains the functional stoma.

12. *Answer:* **D**

    Rationale: The Whipple procedure includes resection of the head of the pancreas, a pancreatojejunostomy, gastrojejunostomy, and vagotomy.

13. After a pancreatectomy, patients may develop steatorrhea, which is characterized by
  A. constipated stool.
  B. mucous stool.
  C. frothy stool with fat particles.
  D. blood in stool.

14. Which type of diet increases the symptoms of dumping syndrome following a gastrectomy?
  A. High fat.
  B. High carbohydrate.
  C. Low protein.
  D. Low fat.

15. In the United States, esophageal cancer is most common in which group?
  A. Native Americans.
  B. Blacks.
  C. Caucasians.
  D. Eastern Europeans.

16. Esophageal cancer most commonly occurs in which section of the esophagus?
  A. Upper thoracic esophagus.
  B. Terminal esophagus.
  C. Lower thoracic esophagus.
  D. Cervical esophagus.

17. The most common site of metastasis in colon cancer is the
  A. lung.
  B. liver.
  C. bone.
  D. brain.

Hematologic and Lymphatic Systems
Cathy Mazzone

Select the BEST answer for all of the following questions:

1. Blood components for patients with immune-deficient malignancies should be irradiated prior to transfusion to prevent
  A. cytomegalovirus exposure.
  B. graft-versus-host-disease.
  C. antibody exposure.
  D. febrile reaction.

2. The patient with multiple myeloma is at high risk for developing all of the following complications **EXCEPT**
  A. infection.
  B. renal failure.
  C. ascites.
  D. hypercalcemia.

3. Complications observed in patients with multiple myeloma are due to
  A. bone marrow involvement and systemic effects of substances secreted by the malignant plasma cells.
  B. increased white blood cell and platelet production.
  C. increased red blood cell and immunoglobulin production.
  D. increased platelet production and bone destruction.

4. The incidence of non-Hodgkin's lymphomas
  A. increases with age and is more common in men.
  B. decreases with age and is more common in men.
  C. decreases with age and is more common in women.
  D. increases with age and is more common in women.

13. *Answer:* **C**

Rationale: These are the defining characteristics of steatorrhea.

14. *Answer:* **B**

Rationale: The recommended diet in the presence of dumping syndrome is low carbohydrate, high protein, and moderate fat.

15. *Answer:* **B**

Rationale: In cancer of the esophagus, the age-adjusted mortality rate per 100,000 is: Black men, 16.4%; Black women, 4.1%; white men, 5.7%; and white women, 1.5%.

16. *Answer:* **C**

Rationale: The distribution of esophageal cancer sites is cervical esophagus, 20%; upper thoracic esophagus, 37%; lower thoracic esophagus, 43%.

17. *Answer:* **B**

Rationale: More than 50% of deaths following surgery for colon cancer are secondary to liver metastasis.

REFERENCES

Boarini J, (1990). Gastrointestinal Cancer: Colon, Rectum and Anus, in, Groenwald SL, Frogge MH, Goodman M, and Yarbro CH, (eds). *Cancer Nursing Principles and Practice*, (2nd ed). Boston: Jones and Bartlett, pp. 792–805.

Brennan M, Linsella T, Friedman M, (1989). Cancer of the Pancreas, in, DeVita VT, Hellman S, Rosenberg S, (eds). *Cancer: Principles and Practice of Oncology*, (3rd ed). Philadelphia: JB Lippincott, p. 806.

Clinical Courier NIH, (1990). *Consensus Development Conference.* 8, (10), ISSN 0264-6684.

Cohen A, Shank B, Friedman M, (1989). Colorectal Cancer, in, DeVita VT, Hellman S, Rosenberg S, (eds). *Cancer: Principles and Practice of Oncology*, (3rd ed). Philadelphia: JB Lippincott, p. 907.

Ehlke G, (1991). Gastrointestinal Cancers, in, Baird SB, McCorkle R, Grant M, (eds). *Cancer Nursing: A Comprehensive Textbook.* Philadephia: WB Saunders, pp. 485–501.

Frogge M, (1990). Gastrointestinal Cancer: Esophagus, Stomach, Liver, and Pancreas, in, Gronewald SL, Frogge MH, Goodman M, Yarbro CH, (eds). *Cancer Nursing Principles and Practice*, (2nd ed). Boston: Jones and Bartlett, pp. 806–844.

Hilderly L, (1990). Radiotherapy, in, Groenwald SL, Frogge MH, Goodman M, Yarbro CH, (eds). *Cancer Nursing Principles and Practice*, (2nd ed). Boston: Jones and Bartlett, pp. 199–231.

Holyoke ED, (1988). The Role of Carcinoembryonic Antigen in the Management of Patients with Colorectal Cancer. *Cancer: Principles and Practice of Oncology Updates.* 2 (3): 1–11.

MacDonald J, (1989). Adjuvant Therapy of Colorectal Cancer: Where Do We Stand? *Oncology.* 3 (6): 87–92.

McNally JC, Somerville ET, Miaskowski C, Rostad M, (eds), (1991). Elimination, in, *Guidelines for Cancer Nursing Practice*, (2nd ed). Philadelphia: WB Saunders. pp. 295–315.

Sarsinero GE, (1991). Knowledge Deficit Related to Prevention and Early Detection of Colorectal Cancer, in, McNally JC, Somerville ET, Miaskowski C, Rostad M, (eds). *Guidelines for Oncology Nursing Practice*, (2nd ed). Philadelphia: WB Saunders, pp. 17–21.

Strohl RA, (1992). Colorectal Cancers, in, Clark JC, McGee RF, (eds). *Core Curriculum in Oncology Nursing*, (2nd ed). Philadelphia: WB Saunders.

Hematologic and Lymphatic Systems

1. *Answer:* **B**

Rationale: Irradiation kills the T cells in the blood component, thus preventing transfusion-related graft-versus-host disease.

2. *Answer:* **C**

Rationale: Ascites is not a complication associated with multiple myeloma.

3. *Answer:* **A**

Rationale: Major complications of multiple myeloma include bone pain, hypercalcemia, renal failure, anemia, and impaired immune responses that are the result of bone marrow involvement and systemic effects of substances secreted by the malignant plasma cells.

4. *Answer:* **A**

Rationale: The average age at diagnosis is 42, and the incidence increases with age. Non-Hodgkin's lymphomas are more common in men.

5. Mr. H has an intensive diffuse histolytic lymphoma involving his abdomen. He is to start chemotherapy today. The nurse should assess for all of the following potential complications **EXCEPT**
   A. tumor lysis syndrome.
   B. gastrointestinal obstruction.
   C. infection.
   D. peripheral neuropathy.

6. An increased incidence of second malignancies has been observed in patients receiving intensive radiation therapy and/or chemotherapy for which malignancy?
   A. Leukemia.
   B. Colon cancer.
   C. Hodgkin's disease.
   D. Breast cancer.

7. Patients with Hodgkin's disease typically may present with any of the following symptoms **EXCEPT**
   A. fever.
   B. sweating.
   C. pruritus.
   D. erythematous rash.

8. The most commonly used chemotherapy protocol for Hodgkin's disease is
   A. nitrogen mustard, vincristine, procarbazine, and prednisone.
   B. nitrogen mustard, velban, daunomycin, and prednisone.
   C. nitrogen mustard, procarbazine, and velban.
   D. nitrogen mustard, etoposide, vincristine, and prednisone.

9. Mrs. H is receiving chemotherapy for acute leukemia. She presents with gait and speech alterations and a decreased ability to perform rapid alternating movements. Which chemotherapeutic agent is responsible for these symptoms?
   A. Daunorubicin.
   B. High-dose cytarabine.
   C. L-asparaginase.
   D. Cytarabine.

10. Patients with acute leukemia are at risk for all of the following treatment complications **EXCEPT**
   A. bleeding.
   B. leukostasis.
   C. infection.
   D. cataracts.

11. Myelodysplastic syndromes can be defined by all of the following characteristics **EXCEPT** that they
   A. are a group of heterogeneous disorders of the blood.
   B. may progress to acute myelogenous leukemia.
   C. are often referred to as preleukemia.
   D. respond well to treatment.

12. Which type of leukemia is treated with prophylactic central nervous system radiation therapy or chemotherapy?
   A. Acute nonlymphocytic leukemia.
   B. Chronic myelogenous leukemia.
   C. Acute lymphocytic leukemia.
   D. Chronic lymphocytic leukemia.

13. Which type of leukemia is associated with an increased risk for disseminated intravascular coagulopathy?
   A. Acute promyelocytic leukemia.
   B. Acute monocytic leukemia.
   C. Chronic lymphocytic leukemia.
   D. Acute myelocytic leukemia.

14. Acute myelogenous leukemia (AML) is also referred to as
   A. acute nonlymphocytic leukemia (ANLL).
   B. acute lymphocytic leukemia (ALL).
   C. myelodysplastic syndrome (MDS).
   D. hairy cell leukemia.

15. Which of the following characteristics **IS NOT** associated with chronic leukemia?
   A. Predominant cell is mature appearing.
   B. Gradual onset of disease.
   C. Rapid disease progression.
   D. Primarily affects older adults.

5. *Answer:* **D**

Rationale: Peripheral neuropathy is not an expected complication in the patient with diffuse histolytic lymphoma.

6. *Answer:* **C**

Rationale: Patients who receive radiation therapy and/or chemotherapy for Hodgkin's disease have an increased incidence of second malignancies.

7. *Answer:* **D**

Rationale: Fever, sweating, pruritus, and weight loss are common symptoms of patients with Hodgkin's disease.

8. *Answer:* **A**

Rationale: The most commonly used chemotherapy protocol for Hodgkin's disease is MOPP consisting of nitrogen mustard, vincristine, procarbazine, and prednisone.

9. *Answer:* **B**

Rationale: Cerebellar and cerebral toxicity can occur with high-dose cytarabine.

10. *Answer:* **D**

Rationale: Patients with acute leukemia are not at risk for the development of cataracts because radiation therapy to the eyes is not part of the treatment plan.

11. *Answer:* **D**

Rationale: Myelodysplastic syndromes are often refractory to treatment and are associated with a poor prognosis.

12. *Answer:* **C**

Rationale: Central nervous system involvement is common in acute lymphocytic leukemia, hence prophylactic treatment with either radiation therapy or chemotherapy is administered.

13. *Answer:* **A**

Rationale: Acute promyelocytic leukemia is associated with an increased risk for the development of disseminated intravascular coagulopathy (DIC). Patients may present with DIC and then be diagnosed with acute promyelocytic leukemia.

14. *Answer:* **A**

Rationale: Acute myelogenous leukemia is also referred to as acute *non*lymphocytic leukemia because the major cell line involved is the myelocyte.

15. *Answer:* **C**

Rationale: Chronic leukemia progresses over a period of years rather than weeks.

16. The initial treatment phase of acute leukemia usually consists of
   A. multiple chemotherapeutic agents administered.
   B. single agent, continuous infusion over five to seven days.
   C. radiation and low-dose chemotherapy.
   D. interferon and chemotherapy in high doses.

17. The requirement for a complete remission in acute leukemia includes all of the following EXCEPT
   A. absence of all clinical signs and symptoms of leukemia.
   B. normal peripheral blood differential devoid of blasts.
   C. restoration of normal bone marrow with <5% blasts.
   D. adequate numbers of maturing blood precursors.

18. Measures the nurse should implement to prevent the development of a perianal infection in the patient with acute leukemia include all of the following EXCEPT
   A. avoid rectal temperatures and suppositories.
   B. encourage friction drying of perianal area.
   C. encourage the patient to go without underwear.
   D. cleanse the area with mild soap and water after every stool.

Skin

Alice J. Longman

Select the BEST answer for all of the following questions:

1. Which of the following is **NOT** a characteristic of malignant melanoma?
   A. Color variegation is apparent in the lesion.
   B. The border of the lesion is irregular.
   C. The lesion is asymmetrical.
   D. The lesion is indurated.

2. What is the single most important factor in the accurate diagnosis of skin cancer?
   A. Assessing the extension into nearby structures.
   B. Leaving a margin to demarcate the lesion.
   C. Obtaining an adequate specimen with margins for accurate diagnosis.
   D. Ensuring acceptable cosmetic results.

3. Which of the following is the major reason for accurate assessment of a suspicious malignant melanoma?
   A. Malignant melanoma has the ability to spread rapidly to other sites of the body.
   B. The level of invasion and tumor thickness is best assessed by microstaging.
   C. Microscopic examination is essential for determination of the exact type of malignant melanoma.
   D. Palliative treatment of malignant melanoma is best achieved by accurate assessment.

4. Which of the standard therapies for the treatment of cancer is most effective in the treatment of skin cancer?
   A. Surgical excision.
   B. Radiation therapy.
   C. Chemotherapy.
   D. Hormonal therapy/biotherapy.

5. Which of the following is **NOT** a reason for using radiotherapy in the treatment of malignant melanoma?
   A. Relief of symptoms is necessary.
   B. The tumor volume is high.
   C. Subcutaneous, cutaneous, or nodal metastases are inaccessible.
   D. Recurrent lesions may be inoperable.

16. *Answer:* **A**

Rationale: The initial treatment phase of acute leukemia consists of multiple chemotherapeutic agents administered to kill (normal and leukemic) hematopoietic cells so that normal marrow elements may repopulate.

17. *Answer:* **D**

Rationale: Remission is defined as the absence of all clinical and microscopic signs of leukemia, return of normal cellularity and hematopoietic elements, and restoration of a normal bone marrow with less than 5% blasts present.

18. *Answer:* **B**

Rationale: Excessive rubbing/friction of perianal area will promote skin breakdown which may result in infection.

REFERENCES

Alexander EJ, (1992). Lymphomas, in, Clark JC, McGee RF, (eds). *Core Curriculum in Oncology Nursing,* (2nd ed). Philadelphia: WB Saunders.

Balz SB, Dodd MJ, Di Juleo JE, (1991). Nursing Management of Persons Treated for Cure: Prototype-Hodgkin's Disease, in, Baird SB, McCorkle R, Grant M, (eds). *Cancer Nursing: A Comprehensive Textbook.* Philadephia: WB Saunders, pp. 673–688.

Carson C, Callaghan MC, (1991). Hematopoietic and Immunologic Cancers, in, Baird SB, McCorkle R, Grant M, (eds). *Cancer Nursing: A Comprehensive Textbook.* Philadephia: WB Saunders, pp. 536–566.

Cook MB, (1990). Multiple Myeloma, in, Groenwald SL, Frogge MH, Goodman M, Yarbro CH, (eds). *Cancer Nursing Principles and Practice,* (2nd ed). Boston: Jones and Bartlett, pp. 990–998.

Maguire-Eisen M, (1990). Diagnosis and Treatment of Adult Acute Leukemia. *Seminars in Oncology Nursing.* 6 (1): 17–24.

Maguire-Eisen M, (1992). Leukemias, in, Clark JC, McGee RF, (eds). *Core Curriculum in Oncology Nursing,* (2nd ed). Philadelphia: WB Saunders.

Newman KA, (1985). The Leukemias. *Nursing Clinics of North America.* 20: 227–234.

Wujcik D, (1990). Leukemia, in, Groenwald SL, Frogge MH, Goodman M, Yarbro CH, (eds). *Cancer Nursing Principles and Practice.* Boston: Jones and Bartlett, pp. 930–947.

Yarbro CH, (1990). Lymphomas, in, Groenwald SL, Frogge MH, Goodman M, Yarbro CH, (eds). *Cancer Nursing Principles and Practice.* (2nd ed). Boston: Jones and Bartlett, pp. 974–989.

Yeomans AC, Harle MT, (1990). Myelodysplastic Syndromes. *Seminars in Oncology Nursing.* 6 (1): 17–24.

Skin

1. *Answer:* **D**

Rationale: Malignant melanoma arises from melanocytes which are important in the transport of melanin. Malignant melanoma is characterized by radial and/or vertical growth. Most melanomas are asymmetrical in appearance because of the tissue from which they arise.

2. *Answer:* **C**

Rationale: To diagnose the exact type of skin cancer, an adequate specimen is most important, therefore excision or punch biopsy is required.

3. *Answer:* **A**

Rationale: Of all the skin cancers, malignant melanoma is the most aggressive and virulent. Those persons at risk for developing malignant melanoma are cautioned to have regular and complete examination of the skin.

4. *Answer:* **A**

Rationale: While all of the standard therapies may be used during the course of treatment for skin cancer, surgical excision is used in 90% of the cases. In the treatment of malignant melanoma, it may be necessary to remove nearby lymph nodes.

5. *Answer:* **B**

Rationale: While surgery is the treatment of choice for malignant melanoma, radiotherapy may be used as adjunct therapy. The indications for the use of radiotherapy are when the tumor volume is low, symptom relief, inoperable recurrent disease, or nodes are inaccessible for surgical relief.

6. Which of the following chemotherapeutic agents has had the most consistent results in the treatment of malignant melanoma?
   A. Nitrosureas (BCNU, CCNU, methyl-CCNU).
   B. Monoclonal antibodies.
   C. Hormonal agents.
   D. Dacarbazine (DTIC).

7. Of the following persons, who would be at the **HIGHEST** risk of developing non-melanoma skin cancer?
   A. A 35-year-old Caucasian ski instructor in the western United States.
   B. A 60-year-old Caucasian grain farmer in the midwestern United States.
   C. A 40-year-old Mexican American ranch hand in the southwestern United States.
   D. A 60-year-old black cotton farmer in the southern United States.

8. Which of the following is the most important in follow-up care for persons who have been treated for skin cancer?
   A. Weekly, systematic self-assessment of the skin for suspicious lesions.
   B. Limiting sun exposure to two hours during the summer months.
   C. Evaluation at regular intervals by a physician and/or nurse.
   D. Use of sunscreens and sunblocks whenever outside during the summer months.

9. Which of the following has the highest risk for recurrence?
   A. Superficial spreading melanoma.
   B. Basal cell carcinoma.
   C. Squamous cell carcinoma.
   D. Nodular melanoma.

10. In teaching about the prevention of skin cancer, the **MAJOR AREAS** to be included initially are
   A. length of exposure to sunlight, use of sunscreen (sun protection factor of 15 or more), use of protective clothing, and use of sunglasses.
   B. time of day during sun exposure, time of year of sun exposure, weather conditions during sun exposure, and recreational activities.
   C. skin type, genetic history, family pedigree about skin cancer, and use of tanning parlors.
   D. skin assessment, effect of altitude during sun exposure, time of year during sun exposure, and time of day of sun exposure.

11. In presenting information on the risks associated with the development of malignant melanoma nurses should target
   A. senior citizens.
   B. mothers of adolescents.
   C. construction workers.
   D. mothers of infants and young children.

12. In counseling patients and families about continued care following treatment for skin cancer, which self-care activity is the **MOST** important?
   A. Monthly self-examination of the skin.
   B. Collecting information about skin cancer from national cancer-related organizations.
   C. Updating family history of skin cancers.
   D. Monitoring site where the lesion occurred.

6. *Answer:* **D**

    Rationale: Treatment for malignant melanoma, other than surgery, remains elusive. Of the chemotherapeutic agents tested and used to date, the most consistently effective one is dacarbazine (DTIC).

7. *Answer:* **B**

    Rationale: A history of exposure to sunlight is important in the assessment of persons presenting with skin cancer. Those at highest risk for the development of skin cancer are Caucasians with a chronic exposure to sunlight.

8. *Answer:* **C**

    Rationale: The importance of continued surveillance cannot be overemphasized. Systematic assessment of the skin at regular intervals by a physician or nurse is important; however, monthly self-assessment of the skin is taught and recommended to those who have had skin cancer.

9. *Answer:* **D**

    Rationale: Equally high cure rates with either surgery or radiation can be achieved for basal cell carcinoma and squamous cell carcinoma. While there is a possibility of recurrence with either one, continued surveillance improves the ability to detect it readily. The most important prognostic feature in malignant melanoma is the size of the lesion at the time of diagnosis. Nodular melanoma has the highest risk of recurrence and metastasis.

10. *Answer:* **A**

    Rationale: Exposure to sunlight should be limited between 10 AM and 3 PM in high sun areas. Sunscreens, with sun protection factor of 15 or more, are recommended with frequent reapplications during prolonged sun exposure. Protective clothing and sunglasses are also recommended during prolonged exposure to sunlight. All of these are important in teaching about the prevention of skin cancer.

11. *Answer:* **D**

    Rationale: There is a possible link between severe sunburn in childhood and the risk of malignant melanoma in later life. Children should be protected from traumatic sunburn, and it is advisable to keep infants out of the sun.

12. *Answer:* **A**

    Rationale: Evaluation at regular intervals by a physician or nurse is important for those who have received treatment for skin cancer. Patients and families are instructed to assume responsibility for their own care. One of the most important activities is to engage in monthly skin self-examination.

13. Of the following activities, which would **NOT** be advisable for a person who has been treated for skin cancer?
    A. Daily swimming in a protected pool.
    B. Attending a tanning parlor weekly.
    C. Playing volleyball on a beach occasionally.
    D. Playing golf in the late afternoon.

14. When using sunscreen, which part of the body is most frequently neglected?
    A. The cheeks.
    B. The hands.
    C. The back of the legs.
    D. The back of the neck.

13.   *Answer:* **B**

Rationale: Regular and prolonged exposure to the sun is not recommended for those who have been treated for skin cancer. Tanning parlors are potentially dangerous for those at risk for developing skin cancer and for those who have been treated for skin cancer and are not recommended.

14.   *Answer:* **D**

Rationale: Most people are conscientious in applying sunscreen on their faces. The one area that many forget is the back of the neck. Often, this area is exposed to the sun for long periods of time.

REFERENCES

American Cancer Society, (1990). *Cancer Facts and Figures—1990*. Atlanta, GA: American Cancer Society.

Balch CM, (1987). Cutaneous Melanoma: A Review of Clinical Management. *Texas Medicine*. 83: 70–78.

Berkman S, (1985). The Skin Remembers. *Cancer News*. 29 (2): 2–4.

Frank-Stromborg M, (1986). The Role of the Nurse in Cancer Detection and Screening. *Seminars in Oncology Nursing*. 11 (3): 191–199.

Fraser MC, McGuire DB, (1984). Skin Cancer's Early Warning System. *American Journal of Nursing*. 84 (10): 1232–1236.

Fraser MC, Tokar I, (1991). Knowledge Deficit Related to Prevention and Early Detection of Skin Cancer, in, McNally JC, Somerville ET, Miaskowski C, Rostad M, (eds). *Guidelines for Oncology Nursing Practice*, (2nd ed). Philadelphia: WB Saunders, pp. 35–43.

Friedman RJ, Rigel DS, Kopf AW, (1985). Early Detection of Malignant Melanoma: The Role of Physician Examination and Self-Examination of the Skin. *CA*. 29 (4): 194–215.

Houghton AN, (1987). A Refresher on Melanoma: Suggestions Towards Prevention: Clues to Early Detection. *Your Patient and Cancer*. Winter: 13–18.

Johnson BL, (1987). Malignant Melanoma, in, Groenwald SL, Frogge MH, Goodman M, Yarbro CH, (eds). *Cancer Nursing Principles and Practice*, (2nd ed). Boston: Jones and Bartlett, pp. 684–692.

Loescher LJ, Booth A, (1990). Skin Cancer, in, Groenwald SL, Frogge MH, Goodman M, Yarbro CH, (eds). *Cancer Nursing Principles and Practice*, (2nd ed). Boston: Jones and Bartlett, pp. 99–1014.

Longman A, (1991). Skin Cancers, in, Baird SB, McCorkle R, Grant M, (eds). *Cancer Nursing: A Comprehensive Textbook*. Philadelphia: WB Saunders, pp. 637–646.

Longman A, (1992). Skin Cancer, in, Clark JC, McGee RF, (eds). *Core Curriculum for Oncology Nursing*, (2nd ed). Philadelphia: WB Saunders.

Owen P, (1991). Skin Integrity, Impairment of, Related to Malignant Skin Lesions, in, McNally JC, Somerville ET, Miaskowski C, Rostad M, (eds). *Guidelines for Oncology Nursing Practice*, (2nd ed). Philadelphia: WB Saunders, pp. 231–235.

Stewart DD, (1987). Indoor Tanning: The Nurse's Role in Preventing Skin Damage. *Cancer Nursing*. 10 (2): 93–99.

Head and Neck

Leonita H. Cutright

Select the BEST answer for all of the following questions:

1. Long-term survival for head and neck cancer patients depends on
    A. stage and anatomical location of disease.
    B. size and type of tumor involved.
    C. the absolute number of positive neck nodes found at the time of resection.
    D. tumor secretion of parathyroid hormone.

2. Mr. S has had a supraglottic laryngectomy. He is ready to start oral feedings. The *best* nursing intervention for Mr. S is to
    A. start with water; assess for nausea and vomiting.
    B. discontinue the nasogastric tube; start on a regular diet.
    C. start with semisolids; stay with the patient to assess for aspiration.
    D. keep the nasogastric tube and trach tube intact. It is too early to start oral feedings.

3. Curative treatment for head and neck cancer includes
    A. surgery and radiation.
    B. radiation and chemotherapy.
    C. chemotherapy and surgery.
    D. biotherapy and surgery.

4. An excisional biopsy of a suspicious neck node is contraindicated except when
    A. lymphoma is suspected.
    B. the surgical risk is too high.
    C. a synchronous primary is suspected.
    D. chemotherapy is not an option.

5. Mr. W has had a total laryngectomy and right radical neck dissection. The final pathology report indicates that three nodes were positive. Which treatment plan is most likely to be recommended?
    A. No further treatment.
    B. Postop radiation over a four- to six-week period.
    C. Adjuvant chemotherapy for six months.
    D. Further surgery to implant I-125 seeds in the neck.

6. Mr. C is three days postop composite neck resection with reconstruction using a pectoralis major myocutaneous flap. He seems depressed and withdrawn. The most appropriate nursing intervention to facilitate initial adjustment would be to
    A. initiate a consult.
    B. encourage self-care activities.
    C. give him a mirror.
    D. tell him he doesn't look too bad.

7. The most common site for development of head and neck cancer is the
    A. oral cavity.
    B. maxillary sinus.
    C. nasopharynx.
    D. larynx.

8. A patient is diagnosed with a T3, N1, M0 squamous cell carcinoma of the right tonsil. The treatment for this disease is
    A. surgery and chemotherapy.
    B. radiation alone.
    C. surgery and radiation.
    D. radiation and chemotherapy.

9. Which of the following means of providing oral care following head and neck surgery is contraindicated?
    A. Normal saline gavage.
    B. Water Pic.
    C. Mechanically removing crusts.
    D. Lemon-glycerin swabs.

1. *Answer:* **A**

    Rationale: Survival rate depends on the specific anatomical location of the primary tumor and stage of the disease at the time of diagnosis.

2. *Answer:* **C**

    Rationale: Patients who have had a supraglottic laryngectomy are prone to aspiration until they learn new swallowing techniques. Semisolids are best to start oral intake. Water and thin liquids are the last substances these patients learn to swallow. The nasogastric tube should be maintained to provide adequate nutrition until adequate oral intake is achieved.

3. *Answer:* **A**

    Rationale: Surgery or radiation alone is used for Stage I and II cancers of the head and neck. Surgery and radiation in combination are used for stage III and IV disease. Chemotherapy is used primarily as palliative treatment. Biotherapy is only used experimentally.

4. *Answer:* **A**

    Rationale: An excisional biopsy is done when non-otolaryngologists are working up a patient with a suspicious neck node. An excisional biopsy can lead to seeding of the tumor. This can increase the incidence of tumor recurrence.

5. *Answer:* **B**

    Rationale: External beam-radiation is given over a four- to six-week period in the postop head and neck patient with positive lymph nodes. The dosage of approximately 5000 rads is to ensure eradication of micrometastasis.

6. *Answer:* **B**

    Rationale: Self-care activities are the best way to help the patient cope with changes in appearance and to refocus on normalcy.

7. *Answer:* **A**

    Rationale: The oral cavity comes into frequent contact with environmental carcinogens.

8. *Answer:* **C**

    Rationale: A T3, N1, M0 of the tonsil is a stage IV lesion. This stage is treated with combination therapy—surgery and radiation. Surgery removes the tumor bulk and radiation removes micrometastasis.

9. *Answer:* **D**

    Rationale: Lemon-glycerin swabs have a drying effect on the oral mucosa and have a high sugar content, increasing the opportunity for bacterial growth in the oral cavity.

10. Risk factors for head and neck cancer include all of the following **EXCEPT**
   A. smoking.
   B. alcohol consumption.
   C. high-fat diet.
   D. Epstein-Barr virus.

11. Mr. B is treated surgically for a T3, N1, M0 of the true vocal cord. The resulting dysfunction includes all of the following **EXCEPT**
   A. aphonia.
   B. permanent tracheal stoma.
   C. inability to blow out candles on a birthday cake.
   D. raspy voice.

12. Mr. J returns for his first office visit after a right composite neck resection. He complains of right shoulder pain and a range of motion (ROM) of 90°. An appropriate nursing action is to
   A. obtain a shoulder x-ray for a suspected lytic lesion in the shoulder.
   B. immobilize the arm and shoulder in a sling.
   C. obtain a physical therapy consult for shoulder exercises.
   D. give him a steroid injection in the shoulder.

13. All of the following are late signs of oral cancer **EXCEPT**
   A. trismus.
   B. referred otalgia.
   C. dysphagia.
   D. erythroplakia.

14. Mr. S is five days past a supraglottic laryngectomy and right radical neck dissection. He has a temperature of 100° F and erythema and fluctuance at the suture line. You would
   A. keep the patient on bedrest, prepare carotid blow out kit, and call the OR alerting them to an impending carotid rupture.
   B. continue nasogastric tube (NGT) feedings and perform dressing changes as needed.
   C. administer IV antibiotics to treat aspiration pneumonia.
   D. begin oral feedings and discontinue the nasogastric tube.

10. *Answer:* **C**

Rationale: Smoking and alcohol consumption are the classic risk factors for cancers of the oral cavity, oropharynx, and larynx. The Epstein-Barr virus is associated with cancers of the nasopharynx. A high-fat diet has not been identified as a risk factor for head and neck cancers.

11. *Answer:* **D**

Rationale: Surgical treatment of a T3, N1, M0 of the true vocal cords requires a total laryngectomy. Resulting dysfunction includes loss of voice (aphonia), permanent tracheal stoma, and no air source from the lungs to the mouth. Thus, one is unable to blow out candles on a birthday cake. A supraglottic laryngectomy would result in a raspy voice and some degree of aspiration initially. Differentiating the anatomical changes and resulting dysfunction between a supraglottic and total laryngectomy is required.

12. *Answer:* **C**

Rationale: A composite resection includes a neck dissection with resultant shoulder droop and forward curvature of the spine. Physical therapy for ROM and resistive exercises are the best initial treatment to restore function and decrease pain.

13. *Answer:* **D**

Rationale: Erythroplakia has been shown to be the most common presentation of early cancer. "Despite evidence that leukoplakia is overrated as a clinically significant pathologic entity and has only a low malignant potential, the concept that white lesions of the oral mucosa are precancerous or early carcinoma still abounds in the literature and in teaching institutions" (Mashberg and Samit; 1989).

14. *Answer:* **B**

Rationale: The symptoms presented are consistent with fistula formation, a common complication following head and neck surgery. This is treated conservatively with dressing changes and NGT feedings.

15.   Prior to receiving external beam-radiation for cancer in the floor of mouth, which consult is mandatory?

    A. Medical oncology.
    B. Physical therapy.
    C. Social services.
    D. Dental service.

16.   The primary cause of death in patients with head and neck cancer is

    A. lung metastasis.
    B. local/regional disease.
    C. liver metastasis.
    D. carotid bleed.

15. *Answer:* **D**

Rationale: The loss of saliva that results from radiation to the oral cavity may lead to dental caries. Meticulous oral hygiene and prophylactic dental care are essential components of the radiation treatment plan.

16. *Answer:* **B**

Rationale: Head and neck tumors act differently from many cancers. This is a locally aggressive disease and must be recognized and treated as such.

REFERENCES

Adams GL, (1989). Malignant Tumors of the Head and Neck, in, Adams GL, et al., (eds). *Fundamentals of Otolaryngology*, (6th ed). Philadelphia: WB Saunders, p. 459.

Cancer Facts and Figures, (1990). Atlanta, GA: American Cancer Society.

Cohen JI, (1989). Benign Neck Masses, in, Adams GL, et al., (eds). *Fundamentals of Otolaryngology*, (6th ed). Philadelphia: WB Saunders, p. 437.

Cutright LH, (1992). Head and Neck Cancer, in, Clark JC, McGee RF, (eds). *Core Curriculum for Oncology Nursing,* (2nd ed). Philadelphia: WB Saunders.

Dropkin MJ, Scott DW, (1983). Body Image Reintegration and Coping Effectiveness after Head and Neck Surgery. *Journal of Specialist Otorhinolaryngology Head and Neck Nurses*. 2: 7–16.

Dropkin MJ, (1989). Coping with Disfigurement and Dysfunction after Head and Neck Cancer Surgery: A Conceptual Framework. *Seminars in Oncology Nursing*. 5 (3): 213–219.

Hilderly LJ, (1990). Radiotherapy, in, Groenwald SL, Frogge MH, Goodman M, Yarbro CH, (eds). *Cancer Nursing Principles and Practice*, (2nd ed). Boston: Jones and Bartlett, pp. 199–229.

Goodman M, (1990). Head and Neck Cancer, in, Groenwald SL, Frogge MH, Goodman M, Yarbro CH, (eds). *Cancer Nursing Principles and Practice*, (2nd ed). Boston: Jones and Bartlett, pp. 889–929.

Hannon LM, (1989). Cancer of the Oral Cavity. *Seminars in Oncology Nursing*. 5 (3): 150–159.

Logemann JA, (1989). Swallowing and Communication Rehabilitation. *Seminars in Oncology Nursing*. 5 (3): 205–212.

Mahon SM, (1987). Nursing Interventions for the Patient with a Myocutaneous Flap. *Cancer Nursing*. 10 (1): 21–31.

Mashberg A, Samit AM, (1989). Early Detection, Diagnosis, and Management of Oral and Oropharyngeal Cancer. *CA*. 39 (2): 67–88.

Million RR, Cassisi NJ, Clark JR, (1989). Cancer of the Head and Neck, in, DeVita VT, Hellman S, Rosenberg S, (eds). *Cancer Principles and Practice of Oncology*, (3rd ed). Philadelphia: JB Lippincott, pp. 488–590.

Reese JL, (1991). Head and Neck Cancers, in, Baird SB, McCorkle R, Grant M, (eds). *Cancer Nursing: A Comprehensive Textbook*. Philadephia: WB Saunders, pp. 567–583.

Rice DH, Spiro RH, (1989). *Current Concepts in Head and Neck Cancer*. New York: The American Cancer Society.

Schleper JR, (1991). Knowledge Deficit Related to Prevention and Early Detection of Head and Neck Cancers, in McNally JT, Somerville ET, Miaskowski C, Rostad M, (eds). *Guidelines for Oncology Nursing Practice*, (2nd ed). Philadelphia: WB Saunders, pp. 22–26.

Schoeper JR, (1989). Prevention, Detection, and Diagnosis of Head and Neck Cancer. *Seminars in Oncology Nursing*. 5 (3): 139–141.

Schwartz SS, Yuska CM, (1989). Common Patient Care Issues Following Surgery for Head and Neck Cancer. *Seminars in Oncology Nursing*. 5 (3): 193–194.

Sigler BA, (1989). Care of Patients with Laryngeal Carcinoma. *Seminars in Oncology Nursing*. 5 (3): 160–163.

Strohl RA, (1989). Radiation Therapy for Head and Neck Cancers. *Seminars in Oncology Nursing*. 5 (3): 166–173.

Neurologic

Betty M. Owens

Select the BEST answer for all of the following questions:

1. Which of the following is **NOT** a common symptom exhibited by a patient with a brain tumor?
   A. Excessive sleepiness.
   B. Vomiting.
   C. Fever.
   D. Irritability.

2. Which of the following statements is **TRUE** regarding high-grade astrocytomas?
   A. They metastasize frequently to liver and/or lungs.
   B. They infiltrate into surrounding brain tissue.
   C. They are usually well encapsulated.
   D. They respond well to standard chemotherapy.

3. A lumbar puncture, to assist in diagnosing a brain tumor, is performed for any of the following reasons **EXCEPT** to
   A. assess for malignant cells in the cerebrospinal fluid (CSF).
   B. assess for increased intracranial pressure.
   C. assess for red and white blood cells.
   D. assess for elevated protein.

4. The principle reason cerebral angiography is performed prior to craniotomy for tumor removal is which of the following?
   A. Assist surgeon to plan a surgical approach based on tumor blood supply.
   B. Assess patient's ability to withstand the surgical procedure.
   C. Determine if the tumor is cystic.
   D. Determine if vasospasm is present.

5. CT scan and magnetic resonance imaging (MRI) of the head may be done before and after the intravenous injection of a contrast agent. The injection of the contrast agent usually provides which information not available from films done without contrast?
   A. Extent of edema surrounding the tumor.
   B. Clear enhancement of tumor tissue.
   C. Evidence of hemorrhage into the tumor.
   D. Evidence of hydrocephalus.

6. A young boy, age 6, presents with symptoms of increased intracranial pressure. A subsequent MRI of the head reveals a large cerebellar mass arising from the fourth ventricle. Surgical removal of the mass confirms medulloblastoma. Which staging test is most appropriate for this patient?
   A. Skull x-rays.
   B. Cerebral angiogram.
   C. MRI of the spine.
   D. CT of the head.

7. Which of the following is the *most effective group* of standard chemotherapeutic agents for high-grade gliomas?
   A. Tumor antibiotics.
   B. Nitrosoureas.
   C. Plant alkaloids.
   D. Alkylating agents.

8. A 45-year-old female attorney presents with minor expressive aphasia and papilledema. MRI of the head shows a large mass with the radiographic appearance of a glioblastoma multiformae. The *first step* of the treatment plan would most likely be which of the following?
   A. Stereotactic biopsy only.
   B. No biopsy; radiation only.
   C. Craniotomy for biopsy and gross total resection.
   D. Craniotomy for biopsy and conservative debulking.

1. *Answer:* **C**

   Rationale: Excessive sleepiness, vomiting, and irritability are all symptoms of increased intracranial pressure. Fever is not a symptom of a brain tumor but, instead, may be a symptom of any number of illnesses, including an infectious process in the brain.

2. *Answer:* **B**

   Rationale: High grade astrocytomas infiltrate surrounding brain tissue and are not usually encapsulated. Often they are cystic and may be multicentric on imaging. They rarely metastasize outside of the central nervous system. Standard chemotherapy drugs do not cross the blood-brain barrier.

3. *Answer:* **C**

   Rationale: A lumbar puncture can measure the pressure within the head and may indicate pressure from a brain tumor in a suspected case. The CSF fluid can be analyzed to determine if any malignant cells are present. Protein in the CSF is elevated in one-third of patients with a brain tumor. The fluid can also be tested for RBCs and WBCs but the presence of these is not diagnostic of a brain tumor.

4. *Answer:* **A**

   Rationale: When cerebral angiography is performed in preparation for the surgical resection of a brain tumor, the purpose is to assist the surgeon to plan his surgical approach in order to avoid injuring important blood vessels which may cause hemorrhage or stroke. Angiography does not measure the patient's ability to withstand surgery. CT scan and/or MRI will often reveal cystic areas; angiography will not add to this information. Vasospasm is a problem that occurs with aneurysms that have hemorrhaged but not with brain tumors.

5. *Answer:* **B**

   Rationale: Tumor or abnormal tissue usually can be seen more clearly after the intravenous injection of a contrast agent. Edema and hemorrhage are often evident in a noncontrast scan. Hydrocephalus is evident in a noncontrast scan; this is noted by the size of the ventricles.

6. *Answer:* **C**

   Rationale: Medulloblastoma often seeds down the spinal cord. MRI of the spine and/or a CT myelogram will reveal any metastases. Skull x-rays will provide no further information. An angiogram is only indicated when it is necessary to note the blood flow to the area.

7. *Answer:* **B**

   Rationale: Most chemotherapeutic agents do not cross the blood–brain barrier except for the nitrosoureas. Carmustine (BCNU) and lomustine (CCNU) have been extensively tested, and although they are the most effective, their therapeutic response is still minimal.

8. *Answer:* **D**

   Rationale: In evaluating this patient, the surgeon not only considers the best chance for survival, but also considers the quality of life the patient will have after surgery; therefore, the surgeon will debulk as much tumor as possible without risking permanent speech problems.

9. A 55-year-old male with a three-year history of prostate cancer is admitted through the emergency room after an acute onset of difficulty in walking and a two- to three-week history of back pain. A CT myelogram indicates a partial block at T9 by a probable metastatic tumor. The **MOST APPROPRIATE** treatment regimen for this patient is
   A. decompressive laminectomy followed by radiation therapy.
   B. radiation therapy only.
   C. decompressive laminectomy followed by chemotherapy.
   D. chemotherapy only.

10. Median survival for a patient diagnosed with a glioblastoma multiformae, who had surgery, radiation, and standard chemotherapy, is which of the following?
   A. six to nine months.
   B. twelve to eighteen months.
   C. twenty-four to thirty months.
   D. thirty-six to forty-two months.

11. Of the following, which newly diagnosed brain tumor patient has the **BEST** prognosis?
   A. A 60-year-old with no neurological deficits with a right temporal grade II astrocytoma.
   B. A 21-year-old with no neurological deficits with a right frontal glioblastoma multiformae.
   C. A 40-year-old with no neurological deficits with a brainstem grade II astrocytoma.
   D. A 71-year-old with a left visual field defect with a right occipital anaplastic astrocytoma.

12. Which of the following is the **MOST IM-PORTANT** assessment in planning the care for a hospitalized patient with a brain tumor?
   A. Patient and family coping ability.
   B. Patient and family understanding of diagnosis.
   C. Baseline temperature.
   D. Baseline neurological status.

13. Six hours post-craniotomy, the patient's intracranial pressure (ICP) reading is 22 mm/Hg. What independent nursing action may the nurse immediately take to attempt to reduce the ICP to less than 20 mm/Hg?
   A. Administer 10 mg of dexamethasone IV push.
   B. Irrigate the ventriculostomy with 2 cc of normal saline.
   C. Elevate the head of the bed to 30°.
   D. Administer 50 gms of mannitol IV over 30 min.

14. A 55-year-old male with a history of prostate cancer is admitted with a partial spinal cord block at T11. Which nursing actions are **NOT** appropriate for this patient?
   A. Assess sensation every four hours.
   B. Assess bladder for retention every four hours.
   C. Assess pupillary response every four hours.
   D. Assess motor strength every four hours.

15. A 36-year-old patient with a brain tumor has periods when his seizures are not well controlled. Which of the following is **NOT** an appropriate self-care action?
   A. Reduce his alcohol intake.
   B. Reduce job/family stress.
   C. Increase the dosage of his seizure medication.
   D. Increase daily periods of rest/sleep.

9.   *Answer:* **A**

Rationale: If no motor weakness is present, then the tumor is treated with radiation alone. If motor weakness is present and progressing, a decompressive laminectomy is first necessary to prevent permanent paralysis. Chemotherapy may be effective, but does not work quickly enough to be a first line of treatment in this case.

10.   *Answer:* **B**

Rationale: With surgery alone, survival for a patient with a glioblastoma multiformae is fourteen weeks. With the addition of standard radiation therapy, survival extends to forty to sixty weeks. With the addition of standard chemotherapy, survival can be extended in some cases to eighteen months. Average survival is twelve to eighteen months.

11.   *Answer:* **A**

Rationale: Four factors affecting prognosis in order of priority are listed below:

1.   Histology—low grade a better prognosis.
2.   Tumor location—tumors located in silent/benign areas have a better prognosis.
3.   Clinical/neurological status—patients presenting with no or few deficits do better than patients with many deficits.
4.   Age—younger patients do better than older patients.

A is correct because this patient has a low-grade tumor in a silent area of the brain with no neurological deficits. Although he is 60 years of age (older than the 21- and 40-year-olds), the age factor is less significant than histology or location.

12.   *Answer:* **D**

Rationale: A baseline assessment of the neurological status must be made so that any deviation may be noted. The neurological status of a patient with a brain tumor may change

very slowly or very rapidly and, thus, for the safety of the patient, the most important assessment to be made is the patient's neurological status. The other assessments also are needed to plan the care of the patient, but are not the most important.

13.   *Answer:* **C**

Rationale: Of the listed actions, the only action that is an independent nursing action is elevating the head of the bed to aid in drainage of blood from the brain. Mannitol and dexamethasone may lower the patient's ICP, but require a physician's order to implement. Nurses do not irrigate a ventriculostomy.

14.   *Answer:* **C**

Rationale: Bladder dysfunction and any deterioration in motor strength and/or sensation in a patient with a partial spinal cord block must be immediately reported to the physician—emergency surgical intervention may be indicated. Assessing pupillary response is not a critical nursing action for a patient with a spinal cord problem. Pupillary response is more indicative of a problem within the head.

15.   *Answer:* **C**

Rationale: Patients with brain tumors often experience seizures due to brain injury from the tumor itself or the subsequent treatment modalities. Usually medication is sufficient to control the seizures, but life-style, too, can affect seizure activity. Alcohol, physical exhaustion, and physical and emotional stress can lower the seizure threshold. Medication may need to be adjusted, but must be monitored by a physician, who will check drug blood levels and then order the needed increase or decrease in dosage. The patient himself should not increase the dosage of his seizure medication without instructions from his physician.

16.   A patient with a brain tumor, status postsurgery and cranial irradiation, is left with a visual field defect, short-term memory problem, and seizure problem. Which of the following concerns should be the **FIRST** focus of his rehabilitation?
    A.   Employment concerns.
    B.   Safety concerns.
    C.   Personality change.
    D.   Family role changes.

17.   Coordination with which agency is imperative for the rehabilitation of the pediatric brain tumor patient?
    A.   Social services.
    B.   School system.
    C.   Home health agency.
    D.   Outpatient physical therapy.

16.   *Answer:* **B**

Rationale: Safety issues are a concern in all of the patient's known deficits. Safety must be the first focus of the family to protect the patient from injury. Other concerns, although bothersome, must be secondary.

17.   *Answer:* **B**

Rationale: A concern for the child with a brain tumor is the effect that the brain tumor and subsequent treatment has on the child's development—cognitive, social, psychological, and sexual. Rehabilitation requires close interaction by parents and the health care team with the child's teacher and the school system. The other agencies listed may or may not need to be involved in the rehabilitation, depending on the particular child.

REFERENCES

Bonner K, Siegel K, (1988). Pathology, Treatment and Management of Posterior Fossa Brain Tumors in Childhood. *Journal of Neuroscience Nursing*. 20 (2): 84–93.

Cammermeyer M, Appledorn C, (eds), (1990). *Core Curriculum for Neuroscience Nursing*, (3rd ed). Chicago: American Association of Neuroscience Nurses.

Ciric I, Rovin R, Cozzens J, Eller T, Vick N, Mikael M, (1990). Role of Surgery in the Treatment of Malignant Cerebral Gliomas, in, Apuzzo MJ, (ed). *Malignant Cerebral Glioma*. Park Ridge, IL: American Association of Neurological Surgeons, pp. 141–155.

Gentzsck P, (1991). Mobility, Impaired Physical, Related to Spinal Cord Compression, in, McNally JC, Somerville ET, Miaskowski C, Rostad M, (eds). *Guidelines for Oncology Nursing Practice*, (2nd ed). Philadelphia: WB Saunders, pp. 259–266.

Hickey J, (1986). *The Clinical Practice of Neurological and Neurosurgical Nursing*, (2nd ed). Philadelphia: JB Lippincott.

Mahey C, Mettlin C, Natarajan N, Laws E, Peace B, (1989). National Survey of Patterns of Care for Brain-tumor Patients. *Journal of Neurosurgery*. 71: 826–836.

Osborn A, (1980). *Introduction to Cerebral Angiography*. Philadelphia: Harper and Row.

Owens B, (1992). Neurological Cancer, in, Clark JC, McGee RF, (eds). *Core Curriculum for Oncology Nursing*, (2nd ed). Philadelphia: WB Saunders.

Robinson CR, Ray SC, Seager ML, (1991). Central Nervous System Tumors, in, Baird SB, McCorkle R, Grant M, (eds). *Cancer Nursing: A Comprehensive Textbook*. Philadephia: WB Saunders, pp. 608–636.

Rowland LP, (ed), (1989). *Merritt's Textbook of Neurology*. Philadelphia: Lea and Febiger.

Shiminski-Maher T, (1990). Brain Tumors in Childhood: Implications for Nursing Practice. *Journal of Pediatric Health Care*. 4 (3): 122–130.

Wegmann J, Hakius P, (1990). Central Nervous System Cancers, in, Groenwald SL, Frogge MH, Goodman M, Yarbro CH, (eds). *Cancer Nursing Principles and Practice*, (2nd ed). Boston: Jones and Bartlett, pp. 751–773.

Sarcoma

Tracy Kresek

Select the BEST answer for all of the following questions:

1. The most common body part in which soft tissue sarcoma develops is the
   A. retroperitoneal cavity.
   B. trunk.
   C. extremity.
   D. head and neck.

2. Mr. B is a 47-year-old male who was recently diagnosed with a large (> 10 cm) high-grade sarcoma of the thigh. Which test should be ordered to evaluate the extent of his disease?
   A. Bone scan.
   B. Chest CT.
   C. Head CT.
   D. Abdominal CT.

3. Which technique should be used in order to obtain the most reliable diagnosis in soft tissue sarcoma?
   A. Fine needle aspiration.
   B. Needle biopsy.
   C. Excisional biopsy.
   D. Incisional biopsy.

4. Mr. V has a high-grade, 8 cm mass in his left upper thigh. His surgeon feels he will be able to remove the mass with a limb-sparing operation. The standard treatment for his tumor would be
   A. preop chemotherapy and surgery plus radiation.
   B. surgery alone.
   C. surgery plus radiation.
   D. surgery plus radiation and postop chemotherapy.

5. The single most active chemotherapy for the treatment of soft tissue sarcoma is
   A. cytoxan.
   B. adriamycin.
   C. methotrexate.
   D. dacarbazine.

6. Approximately 80% of all soft tissue sarcomas excised by surgery alone that recur locally will do so within
   A. six months.
   B. twelve months.
   C. twenty-four months.
   D. thirty-six months.

7. In a leiomyosarcoma of the retroperitoneal area, the most common site of *first* metastasis is
   A. bone.
   B. lymph node.
   C. liver.
   D. brain.

8. Mr. M is a 62-year-old male who is ten days postop from a hip arthroplasty for a femoral sarcoma. Discharge teaching should include avoidance of all activities **EXCEPT**
   A. bending over in bed to pull up his sheets.
   B. bending over to pick up an object off the floor.
   C. crossing his legs.
   D. sitting on a hard surface.

1. *Answer:* **C**

Rationale: Sarcoma is a malignant tumor arising from connective tissue. Soft tissue sarcomas arise from connective tissue other than bone.

2. *Answer:* **B**

Rationale: The most common site of metastasis for extremity sarcoma is the lungs. Therefore, a chest CT would be most appropriate.

3. *Answer:* **D**

Rationale: Fine needle aspiration and biopsy do not give enough material for full evaluation (i.e., special stains). An excisional biopsy is only a "shell out" and would necessitate another operation to achieve adequate margins. An incisional biopsy removes a generous portion of tissue which is minimally manipulated.

4. *Answer:* **C**

Rationale: The value of adjuvant chemotherapy for the treatment of high-grade sarcoma of the extremity remains controversial and should be administered only in the context of an investigational trial. Radiation therapy is added to the surgical limb-sparing procedure in order to increase local control.

5. *Answer:* **B**

Rationale: Adriamycin is the most active single agent in the treatment of sarcomas with a response rate of 15% to 35% in various trials.

6. *Answer:* **C**

Rationale: If there is a local recurrence, statistically it will occur 80% of the time within two years of the primary surgery.

7. *Answer:* **C**

Rationale: Retroperitoneal/abdominal sarcomas tend to metastasize to the liver first. They tend to have a more locoregional spread of the disease.

8. *Answer:* **D**

Rationale: Maximum hip flexion should not exceed 70°, and this precaution must be adhered to for approximately two to three months. Sitting on a hard surface should be encouraged for support and proper alignment.

REFERENCES

Blum RLT, (1975). An Overview of Studies with Adriamycin (NCC 123127) in the United States. *Cancer Chemotherapy Report*. 6: 247–251.

Borden EC, Amoto D, Enterline HT, et al., (1983). Randomization Comparison of Adriamycin Regimes for the Treatment of Metastatic Soft Tissue Sarcoma. *Proceedings AACR and ASCO* (abst). C: 902.

Cancer Statistics, (1986). *CA*. 36 (1): 16–17.

Cantin J, McNeer GP, Chu FC, et al., (1968). The Problem of Local Recurrence after Treatment of Soft Tissue Sarcoma. *Annals of Surgery*. 168: 47–53.

Chang AE, Rosenberg SA, (1988). Clinical Evaluation and Treatment of Soft Tissue Tumors, in, Enzinger FM, Weiss SW, (eds). *Soft Tissue Tumors*, (2nd ed). St. Louis: CV Mosby Co., pp. 19–42.

Chang AE, Rosenberg SA, Glatstein EJ, Antman KA, (1989). Sarcomas of Soft Tissue, in, DeVita VT, Hellman S, Rosenberg S, (eds). *Cancer Principles and Practice of Oncology*, (3rd ed). Philadelphia: JB Lippincott, pp. 1345–1398.

Huth JF, Eilber FR, (1988). Patterns of Metastatic Spread Following Resection of Extremity Soft Tissue Sarcomas and Strategies for Treatment. *Seminars in Surgical Oncology*. 4: 20–26.

Kaiser J, (1986). Hip Arthroplasty for Pathological Fracture, in, Brown MH, Kiss ME, Outlaw E, Viamontes CM, (eds). *Standards of Oncology Nursing Practice*. New York: John Wiley and Sons, pp. 375–389.

Kaiser J, Ross NJ, Piasecke PA, Thorp DM, (1986). Oncology, in, Pellino TA, Mooney NE, Salmond SW, Veradisco LA, (eds). *NOAN Core Curriculum for Orthopedic Nursing*. Pitman: Anthony J. Jannetti, Inc., pp. 147–161.

McNally JC, Somerville ET, Miaskowski C, Rostad M, (eds). (1991). Mobility, in, *Guidelines for Oncology Nursing Practice*, (2nd ed). Philadelphia: WB Saunders, pp. 257–294.

Rosenberg SA, Suit HD, Baker LH, Rosen G, (1982). Sarcomas of the Soft Tissue and Bone, in, DeVita VT, Hellman S, Rosenberg S, (eds). *Cancer Principles and Practice of Oncology*. Philadelphia: JB Lippincott, pp. 1036–1093.

Shiu MH, Brennan MF, (1989). Biopsy of Soft Tissue Sarcoma, in Shiu MH, Brennan MF, (eds). *Surgical Management of Soft Tissue Sarcoma*. Philadelphia: Lea and Febiger, pp. 58–63.

Smith-Brassards A, (1991). Soft Tissue and Bone Sarcomas, in, Baird SB, McCorkle R, Grant M, (eds). *Cancer Nursing: A Comprehensive Textbook*. Philadelphia: WB Saunders, pp. 597–607.

HIV Infection and AIDS

James P. Halloran

Select the BEST answer for all of the following questions:

1.   Mr. J is a gay male with widely disseminated human immunodeficiency virus (HIV)-related Kaposi's sarcoma, whose death is expected within weeks. He has stated that he has had a strained relationship with his parents for many years and has been in a stable relationship with his lover, Mr. P, for the last eight years. Mr. J and Mr. P have discussed treatment options and are in accord. Mr. J expresses to you his concern that his parents will not honor his wishes regarding his code status. In planning Mr. J's care in this situation, it is important to assess
   A.   the religion of Mr. J's parents.
   B.   the health of Mr. J's siblings.
   C.   Mr. J's insurance coverage for critical care.
   D.   whether Mr. J has executed a durable power of attorney.

2.   Mr. K is a 34-year-old male with a diagnosis of HIV-related primary central nervous system (CNS) lymphoma. He lives alone. In preparing Mr. K to return home, the nurse would instruct him to
   A.   avoid fatty foods.
   B.   keep a written daily schedule of routines and appointments.
   C.   not wash his hair until after his last treatment.
   D.   use only disposable tableware.

3.   Ms. M is a 29-year-old female with HIV disease acquired through sharing equipment to inject IV drugs. She relates a ten-year history of opiate and other substance abuse, but states that she has been drug-free for three months. In planning Ms. M's care, the nurse must keep in mind that
   A.   her history of opiate abuse may indicate a heightened sensitivity to the effects of narcotic analgesics.
   B.   persons with a substance abuse history generally recover more quickly than people who acquired the virus through sexual routes.
   C.   her past opiate abuse may indicate the need for higher dosage of narcotic analgesics due to tolerance.
   D.   Ms. M's probable impaired hepatic function indicates that her body will metabolize analgesics more slowly; thus, she will need less frequent medication.

4.   Treatment of HIV-related lymphoma using an aggressive chemotherapeutic approach
   A.   is associated with longer survival than a more conservative approach.
   B.   is associated with shorter survival than a more conservative approach.
   C.   is usually successful in eradicating extranodal disease.
   D.   appears to decrease the incidence of opportunistic infections.

5.   Mr. L has been recently diagnosed with HIV-related dementia. In preparing Mr. L for discharge, all of the following would be appropriate to include in teaching **EXCEPT** to
   A.   keep clocks, calendars, and nightlights handy.
   B.   restrict social contacts to only members of his immediate family.
   C.   make activity lists.
   D.   keep routines simple and consistent.

1. *Answer:* **D**

    Rationale: The legal determinant of the authority to make decisions regarding care relates to the properly executed power of attorney. With death imminent, it is essential that details regarding the patient's wishes be documented. Because the family may not agree with these wishes, the nurse may assist in honoring the patient's desires by assisting with the execution of a power of attorney by referral to the proper resource.

2. *Answer:* **B**

    Rationale: Persons with CNS lesions are prone to memory lapses. A written record is useful as a reminder of routine tasks and scheduled events. No restriction on dietary fat is required unless indicated by a comorbid condition; hair washing is not contraindicated in chemotherapy patients; and standard household routines are adequate for dishes and tableware used by HIV-infected persons.

3. *Answer:* **C**

    Rationale: Tolerance to the effects of opiates increases with use. Patients who have used opiates regularly in the past may require higher doses of narcotic analgesics with quicker recovery. This may complicate the clinical picture. There is no indication that the route of transmission of HIV relates to prognosis. Persons with a history of IV drug use may have hepatic dysfunction, but this does not reduce the need for medication.

4. *Answer:* **B**

    Rationale: The underlying immune lesion that allows the lymphoproliferative disorder to emerge is not successfully treated with cytotoxic chemotherapy; thus, the disease is not eradicated. Aggressive treatment and attendant iatrogenic myelosuppression in the already immunocompromised host does not prolong, and may even shorten, survival and contribute to development of opportunistic infections.

5. *Answer:* **B**

    Rationale: Environmental cues are helpful in managing the cognitive dysfunction characteristic of HIV-related dementia. Restriction of social contact is not helpful; the mobilization of a social support network is vital in adapting to the limitations of HIV-related illness. Restricting contact would not help accomplish mobilization.

6. Ms. W is a 30-year-old female who has been HIV-positive for three years. Her latest CD4 count is 135. Ms. W was admitted with her first episode of Pneumocystis carinii pneumonia (PCP), which has responded to treatment. Ms. W is returning home. In preparing Ms. W for discharge, the nurse would
   A. advise repeat HIV antibody testing to confirm infection.
   B. instruct Ms. W to avoid sharing eating utensils with family members.
   C. instruct Ms. W to report signs and symptoms of other opportunistic infections.
   D. advise Ms. W to eat only organically grown lettuce.

7. Mr. A is infected with HIV. In discussing modifications in his lifestyle, the nurse instructs Mr. A to always use a latex condom when engaging in sex. Mr. A's wife dislikes condoms because she finds them very dry and they reduce her pleasure. The nurse would advise the use of a condom-compatible lubricant such as
   A. vegetable oil.
   B. baby oil.
   C. petroleum jelly.
   D. water-based preparations.

8. AIDS-related Kaposi's sarcoma (KS) differs from classic KS in that
   A. classic KS is generally seen only in the pediatric population.
   B. there is no characteristic pattern of presentation seen in AIDS-related KS.
   C. lesions associated with classic KS are less than 2 cm diameter.
   D. women do not develop AIDS-related KS.

9. Symptoms associated with primary central nervous system (CNS) AIDS-related lymphoma include all of the following **EXCEPT**
   A. altered mental status.
   B. seizure disorders.
   C. hemiparesis.
   D. oliguria.

10. Definitive diagnosis of HIV-related CNS malignancy is established by
    A. differential diagnosis.
    B. brain biopsy.
    C. CT.
    D. Magnetic resonance imaging (MRI).

11. Behaviors associated with increased risk for HIV infection include
    A. vaginal intercourse using a condom.
    B. sharing equipment for parenteral drug administration.
    C. eating from the same plate as a person who is infected.
    D. administration of myelosuppressive agents.

12. The laboratory determination most frequently used to determine progression of HIV infection is
    A. absolute CD4 T cell count.
    B. absolute neutrophil count.
    C. absolute lymphocyte count.
    D. absolute erythrocyte count.

13. Radiotherapeutic intervention in AIDS-related Kaposi's sarcoma is generally
    A. curative.
    B. palliative.
    C. effective only at high doses.
    D. contraindicated.

14. All of the following are considered appropriate treatment interventions for AIDS-related lymphoma **EXCEPT**
    A. surgery.
    B. chemotherapy.
    C. radiotherapy.
    D. biological response modifiers.

15. The major toxicity associated with the use of the antiretroviral agent zidovudine (AZT) is
    A. eosinophilia.
    B. anemia.
    C. retinitis.
    D. odynophagia.

6. *Answer:* **C**

Rationale: At this stage of the HIV illness spectrum, the emergence of PCP indicates that the damage to the immune system has reached the threshold at which development of significant opportunistic infections is possible. Early reporting of symptoms may allow for earlier, more successful therapeutic intervention. Repeat antibody testing is superfluous at this point. Sharing of eating utensils is not a vector for HIV transmission. HIV-positive persons should avoid organically grown lettuce due to the possible presence of potential pathogens.

7. *Answer:* **D**

Rationale: Lubricants other than water-based may weaken latex condoms, increasing the likelihood of breakage and exposure.

8. *Answer:* **B**

Rationale: Classic KS is generally seen on the lower extremities, usually distal to the knee, typically in elderly males. HIV-related KS can present in virtually any organ system.

9. *Answer:* **D**

Rationale: Oliguria is not caused by a CNS deficit.

10. *Answer:* **B**

Rationale: Definitive diagnosis of malignant disease can only be made through biopsy. In the HIV patient, a number of different pathologic processes can present as space-occupying lesions in the brain.

11. *Answer:* **B**

Rationale: Sharing of equipment for parenteral drug injection establishes a blood-to-blood route for transmission of HIV. Use of a condom for any type of intercourse prevents the exchange of potentially infectious body fluids. Casual transmission through sharing eating utensils has not occurred. Myelosuppressive agents may cause immunosuppression, but are not implicated in HIV transmission.

12. *Answer:* **A**

Rationale: The GP120 epitope of HIV is attracted preferentially to the CD4 surface marker, which is most abundant on the human T cell. Destruction over time of an increasing number of T4 cells is thought to produce the underlying immune deficiency in HIV disease.

13. *Answer:* **B**

Rationale: Kaposi's sarcoma is generally fairly radiosensitive, and temporary relief from unsightly or obstructive lesions can be obtained. Prevention of the development of new lesions, however, is not achieved with radiotherapy.

14. *Answer:* **A**

Rationale: Surgical treatment is contraindicated in the typical presence of disseminated disease associated with AIDS-related lymphoma.

15. *Answer:* **B**

Rationale: Anemia is the most commonly seen side effect of the administration of zidovudine and may require dosage adjustment.

16. Survival in HIV-infected individuals diagnosed with Kaposi's sarcoma, but without other opportunistic infections or malignancies, has been documented to extend up to
    A. six months.
    B. one year.
    C. two years.
    D. three or more years.

16.   *Answer:* **D**

   Rationale: Individuals diagnosed with KS as the single manifestation of HIV disease survive longer than those with multiple opportunistic infections or malignancies.

REFERENCES

Cooke M, (1990). Ethical Issues in Treating Incompetent AIDS Patients, in, Cohen PT, Sande MA, Volberding PA, (eds). *The AIDS Knowledge Base.* Waltham, MA: The Medical Publishing Group.

Dickinson D, Clark CMF, Gonzales-Swafford MJ, (1988). AIDS Nursing Care in the Home, in, Lewis A, (ed). *Nursing Care of the Person with AIDS/ARC.* Rockville, MD: Aspen Publishers, Inc., p. 230.

Fahey JL, Taylor JMG, Detels R, et al., (1990). The Prognostic Value of Cellular and Serological Markers in Infection with HIV-1. *New England Journal of Medicine.* 322: 166–172.

Gill PS, Levine AM, Meyer PR, et al., (1985). Primary Central Nervous System Lymphoma in Homosexual Men. Clinical, Immunologic and Pathologic Features. *American Journal of Medicine.* 78: 742.

Gill PS, Levine AM, Krailo M, et al., (1987). AIDS-related Malignant Lymphoma: Results of Prospective Treatment Trials. *Journal of Clinical Oncology.* 5: 1322–1328.

Halloran JP, Hughes AM, (1991). Knowledge Deficit Related to Prevention and Early Detection of HIV Disease, in, McNally J, Miaskowski C, Rostad M, Somerville E, (eds). *Guidelines for Cancer Nursing Practice*, (2nd ed). Philadelphia: WB Saunders, pp. 47–54.

Halloran J, (1992). HIV-Related Cancer, in, Clark JC, McGee RF, (eds). *Core Curriculum for Oncology Nursing,* (2nd ed). Philadelphia: WB Saunders.

Hughes AM, Schofferman J, (1991). AIDS and the Spectrum of HIV Disease, in, Baird SB, McCorkle R, Grant M, (eds). *Cancer Nursing: A Comprehensive Textbook.* Philadelphia: WB Saunders, pp. 647–664.

Krigel RL, Friedman-Klien A, (1988). Karposi's Sarcoma in AIDS: Diagnosis and Treatment, in, DeVita VT, Hellman S, Rosenberg S, (eds). *AIDS: Etiology, Diagnosis, Treatment, and Prevention*, (2nd ed). Philadelphia: JB Lippincott, pp. 245–262.

Levine AM, (1988). Reactive and Neoplastic Lymphoproliferative Disorders and Other Miscellaneous Cancers Associated with HIV Infection, in, DeVita VT, Hellman S, Rosenberg S, (eds). *AIDS: Etiology, Diagnosis, Treatment and Prevention*, (2nd ed). Philadelphia: JB Lippincott, pp. 263–276.

Lewis A, (1988). *Nursing Care of the Person with AIDS/ARC.* Rockville, MD: Aspen Publishers.

Ling W, Wesson DR, (1990). Drugs of Abuse—Opiates. *Western Journal of Medicine.* 152: 565–572.

Management of HIV Disease: Treatment Team Workshop Handbook. New York: World Health Communication.

McCutchan JA, (1990). Virology, Immunology, and Clinical Course of HIV Infection. *Journal of Consulting and Clinical Psychology.* 58 (1): 5–12.

Moran TA, (1988). Cancer in HIV Infection, in, Gee G, Moran TA, (eds). *AIDS: Concepts in Nursing Practice.* Baltimore: Williams and Wilkins.

Richman DD, Fischl MA, Grieco MH, et al., (1987). The Toxicity of Azodothymidine (AZT) in the Treatment of Patients with AIDS and AIDS-related Complex. *New England Journal of Medicine.* 317: 192–197.

Ungvarski PJ, (1989). AIDS Dementia Complex: Considerations for Nursing Care. *Journal of the Association of Nurses in AIDS Care.* 1 (1): 10–12.

Index

Death. See also *Mortality*.
  causes of, ranking of, 114
Death anxiety. See also *Anxiety*.
  in survivors, 88
Debulking, 131, 132
Decadron (dexamethasone), in antiemetic therapy, 33,
    34
Definitive therapy, 127, 128
Delirium, 44
Dementia, HIV-related, 217, 218
Dental care. See also *Oral care*.
  radiation therapy and, 208
Dependence, difficulties with, 45, 46
  spinal cord compression and, 67, 68
Depression, 21, 22. See also *Antidepressants*.
Dermatitis, weeping, health care workers with, 98
DES (diethylstilbestrol), vaginal cancer and, 15
Descriptive observational study, 111, 112
Desensitization treatment, 23, 24
Desquamating rash, pruritic, interleukin-2 causing,
    154
Developmental level, assessment of, 101, 102
Developmental tasks, difficulty with, 99, 100
  in different stages of adulthood, 101, 102
Dexamethasone (Decadron), in antiemetic therapy,
    33, 34
Diarrhea, cesium-137 implant and, 135, 136
  decrease in, diet for, 47, 48
  drugs causing, 49, 50
  electrolyte imbalance in, 47, 48
  enteral feedings causing, 164
  GVHD causing, 157, 158
  radiation therapy causing, 191, 192
  skin integrity and, 47, 48
  therapy causing, 48, 49, 50, 191, 192
Diazepam (Valium), side effects of, 24
DIC. See *Disseminated intravascular coagulation
    (DIC)*.
Diet. See also *Nutritional support*.
  caloric intake in, 35, 36
  colon cancer and, 13, 14
  erythropoiesis and, 56, 57
  fat in, 13
  fiber in, 13
    constipation and, 47, 48
  for diarrhea minimization, 47, 48
  in dumping syndrome, 193, 194
  in dysphagia, 29, 30
  in esophagitis, 43, 44
  in xerostomia, 35, 36
  meal size in, frequency and, 35, 36
  objectives for, in NCI Year 2000 Dietary
    Objectives, 13, 14
  potassium in, 32
  retinols in, 108
  taste alterations and, 34
  treatment involving, 159, 160, 161, 162
Diethylstilbestrol (DES), vaginal cancer and, 15
Digital rectal examination, in thrombocytopenia, 47,
    48
Diphenhydramine, for extrapyramidal reactions, 32

Discrimination, employment, 85, 86
Disfigurement. See *Body image*.
Dissection, "en bloc," 131, 132
Disseminated intravascular coagulation (DIC), blood
    products in, 161, 162
  cancers associated with, 62
  causes of, 62
  in leukemia, 195, 196
  laboratory findings in, 63, 64
  nursing care in, primary goal of, 64
  pathophysiology of, 64
  septic shock and, 66
  signs and symptoms of, 61, 62
Diuresis, in tumor lysis syndrome prevention, 69,
    70
Dizziness, in cerebral tissue hypoxia, 58
DNA synthesis, cell cycle and, 144, 150
Double-barrel colostomy, 191, 192
Dry mouth, 35, 36
DTIC (dacarbazine), for melanoma, 200
Dumping syndrome, diet and, 193, 194
Dysfunctional grief, 19, 20
Dysgerminoma, radiation sensitivity of, 134
Dyspareunia, radiation therapy causing, 51, 52
Dysphagia, 29, 30
  xerostomia-related, 36
Dyspnea, 55, 56
  lung cancer and, 171. See also *Lung cancer*.
  superior vena cava syndrome and, 67, 68

Echocardiogram, in cardiac tamponade, 61, 62
Ectopic hormone syndrome, 66
Edema, cerebral, 64
    increased intracranial pressure and, 70
  laryngeal, 72
Education. See also *Information*; *Patient education*;
    Public education.
  standards of, 5-10
Ejaculation, abdominoperineal resection and, 52
Elavil (amitriptyline), for nerve pain, 27, 28
Elderly, cancer sites in, 125, 126
  developmental tasks of, 101, 102
  losses in, adjustment to, 102
  myth about, adversely affecting cancer awareness,
    102
  participation of, in screening, 11, 12
Electrolyte imbalances. See also specific imbalance.
  in tumor lysis syndrome, 31, 32, 67, 68
Emergencies, 61-72. See also specific type.
  radiation therapy in, 134
Emesis, 31, 32, 33, 34
  chemotherapeutic agents causing, 33, 34
Emphysema, 171
Employment discrimination, 85, 86
"En bloc" dissection, 131, 132
Encore program, 180
Endometrial cancer, diagnosis of, 185, 186
  presenting symptom in, 184, 185
  prognosis of, 188
  risk factors for, 13, 14
Enteral feedings, 163, 164, 167, 168